Advanced Research in Ischemic Heart Disease

Advanced Research in Ischemic Heart Disease

Edited by **Warren Lyde**

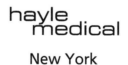

New York

Published by Hayle Medical,
30 West, 37th Street, Suite 612,
New York, NY 10018, USA
www.haylemedical.com

Advanced Research in Ischemic Heart Disease
Edited by Warren Lyde

International Standard Book Number: 978-1-63241-013-9 (Hardback)

Contents

Permissions

List of Contributors

Preface

This book was inspired by the evolution of our times; to answer the curiosity of inquisitive minds. Many developments have occurred across the globe in the recent past which has transformed the progress in the field.

This book encompasses clinical aspects of the management and diagnosis of ischemic heart disease. Ischemic heart disease continues to be a fatal disease with its prevalence across the globe. This book provides an elaborative analysis of ischemic heart disease, including epidemiology, pathogenesis, and diagnostic tests. The aim of this book is to serve as a cutting-edge source of information for the clinical or general researcher, and any clinician involved in the management and diagnosis of this disease. It is basically formulated to fill the vital gap present between these practices and to present a great amalgamation of "fundamentals to bedside and beyond" in the field of ischemic heart disease.

This book was developed from a mere concept to drafts to chapters and finally compiled together as a complete text to benefit the readers across all nations. To ensure the quality of the content we instilled two significant steps in our procedure. The first was to appoint an editorial team that would verify the data and statistics provided in the book and also select the most appropriate and valuable contributions from the plentiful contributions we received from authors worldwide. The next step was to appoint an expert of the topic as the Editor-in-Chief, who would head the project and finally make the necessary amendments and modifications to make the text reader-friendly. I was then commissioned to examine all the material to present the topics in the most comprehensible and productive format.

I would like to take this opportunity to thank all the contributing authors who were supportive enough to contribute their time and knowledge to this project. I also wish to convey my regards to my family who have been extremely supportive during the entire project.

Editor

Part 1

Introduction

Overview of Coronary Artery Disease

Umashankar Lakshmanadoss
Formerly Director, Inpatient Consult Service,
Johns Hopkins University School of Medicine, Baltimore, MD
Division of Cardiology, Guthrie Clinic, Sayre, PA
USA

1. Introduction

Coronary artery disease (CAD) is a major cause of death and disability in developed countries. Although CAD mortality rates have declined over the past four decades in the United States (and elsewhere), CAD remains responsible for about one-third of all deaths in individuals over age 35 [1,2]. It has been estimated that nearly one-half of all middle-aged men and one-third of middle-aged women in the United States will develop some manifestation of CAD.

2. Prevalence

The 2010 Heart Disease and Stroke Statistics update of the American Heart Association reported that 17.6 million persons in the United States have CAD, including 8.5 million with myocardial infarction (MI) and 10.2 million with angina pectoris [2]. The reported prevalence increases with age for both women and men. In a 2009 report that used National Health and Nutrition Examination Survey (NHANES) data, MI prevalence was compared by sex in middle-aged individuals (35 to 54 years) during the 1998 to 1994 and 1999 to 2004 time periods [3]. Although MI prevalence was significantly greater in men than women in both time periods (2.5 versus 0.7 and 2.2 versus 1.0 respectively), there were trends toward a decrease in men and an increase in women. Data from NHANES (and other databases) that rely on self-reported MI and angina from health interviews probably underestimate the actual prevalence of advanced CAD.

This is likely as advanced occlusive coronary artery disease often exists with few symptoms or overt clinical manifestations. Silent ischemia, which is thought to account for 75 percent of all ischemic episodes [4], may be brought to light by electrocardiographic changes (ST segment depression) on an exercise test, ambulatory 24 hour electrocardiographic recording, or periodic routine electrocardiogram (ECG).

3. Global trends

Heart disease mortality has been declining in the United States and in regions where economies and health care systems are relatively advanced, but the experience is often quite different around the world [5]. Coronary artery disease is the number one cause of death in adults from both low- and middle income countries as well as from high-income countries [5]. At the turn of the century, it was reported that CAD mortality was expected to increase approximately 29 percent in women and 48 percent in men in developed countries between 1990 and 2020. The corresponding estimated increases in developing countries were 120 percent in women and 137 percent in men [6].

The most dramatic increments in ischemic heart disease events on a percentage basis were forecast for the Middle East and Latin America. The experience in Asia is especially important because of the large populations involved. In India, CAD may not be largely explained by traditional risk factors [7]. In China, risk factor trends complement tracking of event rates. For example, the dramatic increase in CAD mortality in Beijing is attributable to greater cholesterol levels. The mean cholesterol level was 4.30 mmol/L (166 mg/dL) in 1984 and 5.33 mmol/L (206 mg/dL) only 15 years later [8]. In Latin America, declines in vascular disease rates have been less favorable than in the United States; unfavorable trends in physical activity, obesity, and smoking contribute to these differences [9].

International leaders have called for action plans to avert the projected global epidemic of ischemic heart disease in developing countries [10].

4. Pathophysiology

4.1 Cellular level

Angina is caused by myocardial ischemia, which occurs whenever myocardial oxygen demand exceeds oxygen supply (Figure 1). Because oxygen delivery to the heart is closely

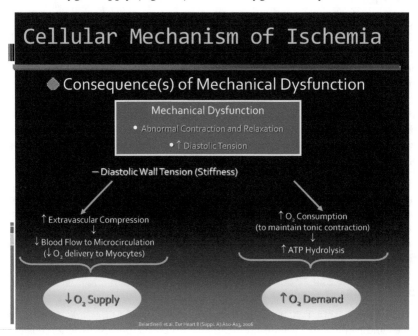

Fig. 1.

coupled to coronary blood flow, a sudden cessation of regional perfusion following a thrombotic coronary occlusion quickly leads to the cessation of aerobic metabolism, depletion of creatine phosphate, and the onset of anaerobic glycolysis. This is followed by the accumulation of tissue lactate, a progressive reduction in tissue ATP levels, and an accumulation of catabolites, including those of the adenine nucleotide pool. As ischemia continues, tissue acidosis develops and there is an efflux of potassium into the extracellular space. Subsequently, ATP levels fall below those required to maintain critical membrane function, resulting in the onset of myocyte death. Irreversible myocardial injury begins after 20 minutes of coronary occlusion in the absence of significant collaterals [11].

Irreversible injury begins in the subendocardium and progresses as a wave front over time, from the subendocardial layers to the subepicardial layers. This reflects the higher oxygen consumption in the subendocardium and the redistribution of collateral flow to the outer layers of the heart by the compressive determinants of flow at reduced coronary pressure. Factors that increase myocardial oxygen consumption (e.g., tachycardia) or reduce oxygen delivery (e.g., anemia, arterial hypotension) accelerate the progression of irreversible injury. In contrast, repetitive reversible ischemia or angina prior to an occlusion can reduce irreversible injury through preconditioning [12].

4.2 Anatomical level

Acute coronary syndrome is usually caused by an unstable atherosclerotic plaque rupture with subsequent platelet-rich thrombus overlying the culprit lesion causing severe narrowing (Figure. 2). This abrupt decrease in blood supply often results in chest pain and ECG changes indicative of ischemia, and, if prolonged, results in myocardial necrosis and

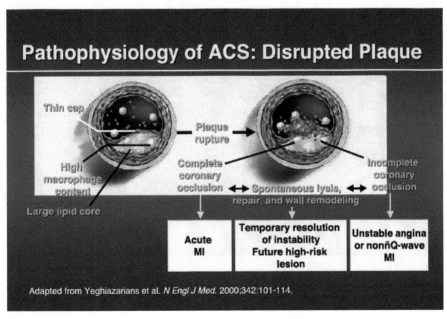

Fig. 2.

enzyme elevation. Less commonly, non ST elevation myocardial infarction is caused by diseases in which myocardial demand exceeds myocardial supply causing a similar clinical presentation. These diseases usually cause a hypermetabolic or high cardiac output state and include hyperthyroidism, anemia, fever, pheochromocytoma, hypertrophic cardiomyopathy, AV fistula and hypertensive urgency/emergency.

Whatever the mechanism of angina may be, patients usually develop the clinical manifestations in a sequence as described in Figure 3. Note that diastolic dysfunction is the earliest manifestation of ischemia, next to perfusion abnormalities which are seen in nuclear studies.

5. Clinical features

Coronary artery disease could be manifesting as a continuum from stable angina to acute coronary syndrome. Angina pectoris is a discomfort in the chest or adjacent areas caused by myocardial ischemia. It is usually brought on by exertion and is associated with a disturbance in myocardial function, without myocardial necrosis.

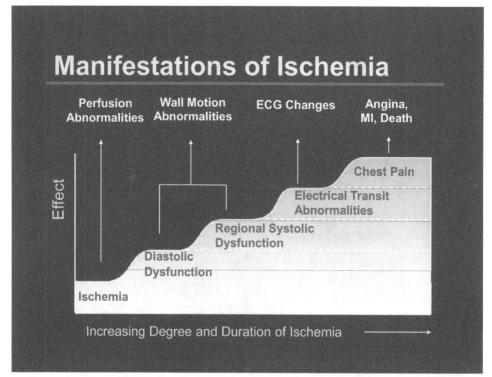

Fig. 3.

Heberden's initial description of angina as conveying a sense of "strangling and anxiety" is still remarkably pertinent. Other adjectives frequently used to describe this distress include viselike, constricting, suffocating, crushing, heavy, and squeezing. In other patients, the quality of the sensation is more vague and described as a mild pressure-like discomfort, an uncomfortable numb sensation, or a burning sensation.

The site of the discomfort is usually retrosternal, but radiation is common and usually occurs down the ulnar surface of the left arm; the right arm and the outer surfaces of both arms may also be involved. Epigastric discomfort alone or in association with chest pressure is not uncommon. Anginal discomfort above the mandible or below the epigastrium is rare. Anginal equivalents (i.e., symptoms of myocardial ischemia other than angina), such as dyspnea, faintness, fatigue, and eructations, are common, particularly in the elderly.

A history of abnormal exertional dyspnea may be an early indicator of CAD even when angina is absent or no evidence of ischemic heart disease can be found on the electrocardiogram (ECG). Dyspnea at rest or with exertion may be a manifestation of severe ischemia, leading to increases in left ventricular (LV) filling pressure. Nocturnal angina should raise the suspicion of sleep apnea.

The term acute coronary syndrome (ACS) is applied to patients in whom there is a suspicion of myocardial ischemia. There are three types of ACS: ST elevation (formerly Q-wave) MI (STEMI), non-ST elevation (formerly non-Q wave) MI (NSTEMI), and unstable angina (UA). The first two are characterized by a typical rise and/or fall in biomarkers of myocyte injury.

For many years, the diagnosis of acute MI relied on the revised criteria established by the World Health Organization (WHO) in 1979. These criteria were epidemiological and aimed at specificity. A joint European Society of Cardiology (ESC) and American College of Cardiology (ACC) committee proposed a more clinically based definition of an acute, evolving, or recent MI in 2000 (13). In 2007 the Joint Task Force of the European Society of Cardiology, American College of Cardiology Foundation, the American Heart Association, and the World Health Federation (ESC/ACCF/AHA/WHF) refined the 2000 criteria and defined acute MI as a clinical event consequent to the death of cardiac myocytes (myocardial necrosis) that is caused by ischemia (as opposed to other etiologies such as myocarditis or trauma) [14].

The criteria used to define MI differ somewhat depending upon the particular clinical circumstance of the patient: those suspected of acute MI based upon their presentation, those undergoing either coronary artery bypass graft surgery or percutaneous intervention, or those who have sustained sudden unexpected, cardiac arrest with or without death [14].

For patients who have undergone recent revascularization or who have sustained cardiac arrest or death, the criteria for the diagnosis of MI are given in detail in the Table 1.

For all other patients in whom there is a suspicion of MI, a typical rise and/or gradual fall (troponin) or more rapid rise and fall (CK-MB) of biochemical markers of myocardial necrosis, with at least one of the following is required:

- Ischemic symptoms
- Development of pathologic Q waves on the ECG
- ECG changes indicative of ischemia (ST segment elevation or depression)
- Imaging evidence of new loss of viable myocardium or a new regional wall motion abnormality.

In addition, pathologic findings (generally at autopsy) of an acute MI are accepted criteria.

The joint task force [14] further refined the definition of MI by developing a clinical classification according to the assumed proximate cause of the myocardial ischemia.

Patulous aneurysmal dilation involving most of the length of a major epicardial coronary artery is present in approximately 1 to 3 percent of patients with obstructive CAD at autopsy or angiography. This angiographic lesion does not appear to affect symptoms, survival, or incidence of MI. Most coronary artery ectasia and/or aneurysms are caused by coronary atherosclerosis (50 percent), and the rest are caused by congenital anomalies and inflammatory diseases, such as Kawasaki disease.

Type 1
Spontaneous myocardial infarction related to ischaemia due to a primary coronary event such as plaque erosion and/or rupture, fissuring, or dissection

Type 2
Myocardial infarction secondary to ischaemia due to either increased oxygen demand or decreased supply, e.g. coronary artery spasm, coronary embolism, anaemia, arrhythmias, hypertension, or hypotension

Type 3
Sudden unexpected cardiac death, including cardiac arrest, often with symptoms suggestive of myocardial ischaemia, accompanied by presumably new ST elevation, or new LBBB, or evidence of fresh thrombus in a coronary artery by angiography and/or at autopsy, but death occurring before blood samples could be obtained, or at a time before the appearance of cardiac biomarkers in the blood

Type 4a
Myocardial infarction associated with PCI

Type 4b
Myocardial infarction associated with stent thrombosis as documented by angiography or at autopsy

Type 5
Myocardial infarction associated with CABG

Table 1. Types of Myocardial Infarction

6. Diagnosis

Evaluation of new onset chest pain in stable individuals should begin with the consideration of imminently life-threatening causes (including acute coronary syndrome, pulmonary embolus, aortic dissection, pneumothorax, and esophageal rupture). This is usually accomplished using clinical judgement, along with ECG testing, and less frequently exercise testing, other noninvasive testing, or invasive angiography.

This is being discussed in detail by other authors in various chapters. nce a life-threatening etiology has been excluded, attempts should be made to identify the specific cause of symptoms and begin treatment. A diagnostic pattern will frequently emerge, based upon the patient's risk factors, description of the pain, and associated symptoms.

Standard clinical characteristics routinely obtained during the initial medical evaluation of patients with UA/NSTEMI can be used to construct a simple classification system that is predictive of risk for death and cardiac ischemic events. The TIMI (Thrombolysis in Myocardial Infarction) risk score (Table 2) includes variables that can be easily ascertained when a patient with UA/NSTEMI presents to the medical care system. The variables used to construct the score were based on observations from prior studies of risk stratification and incorporate demographic and historical features of the patient, measures of the tempo and acuity of the presenting illness, and indicators of the extent of myocardial ischemia and necrosis.

Since patients with an acute coronary syndrome are at increased risk of death and nonfatal cardiac events, clinicians must assess prognosis on an individual basis to formulate plans for evaluation and treatment. The TIMI risk score for UA/NSTEMI is a simple prognostication

TIMI Risk Score	All-Cause Mortality, New or Recurrent MI, or Severe Recurrent Ischemia Requiring Urgent Revascularization Through 14 d After Randomization, %
0–1	4.7
2	8.3
3	13.2
4	19.9
5	26.2
6–7	40.9

The TIMI risk score is determined by the sum of the presence of 7 variables at admission; 1 point is given for each of the following variables:

- age 65 y or older;
- at least 3 risk factors for CAD;
- prior coronary stenosis of 50% or more;
- ST-segment deviation on ECG presentation;
- at least 2 anginal events in prior 24 h;
- use of aspirin in prior 7 d;
- elevated serum cardiac biomarkers.

Prior coronary stenosis of 50% or more remained relatively insensitive to missing information and remained a significant predictor of events.

Table 2. TIMI Risk Score for Unstable Angina/Non-ST Elevation MI

scheme that enables a clinician to categorize a patient's risk of risk of death and ischemic events at the critical initial evaluation. A promising clinical application of this score is identification of a patient for whom new antithrombotic therapies would be especially effective.

While ECG manifestations are an important component of diagnosis, one should be aware of the pitfalls of the ECG. Tables 3, 4 and 5 describe the ECG manifestations of ischemic disease.

ST elevation
New ST elevation at the J-point in two contiguous leads with the cut-off points: ≥ 0.2 mV in men or ≥ 0.15 mV in women in leads V_2–V_3 and/or ≥ 0.1 mV in other leads

ST depression and T-wave changes
New horizontal or down-sloping ST depression ≥ 0.05 mV in two contiguous leads; and/or T inversion ≥ 0.1 mV in two contiguous leads with prominent R-wave or R/S ratio >1

Table 3. ECG manifestations of acute myocardial ischemia (in absence of LVH and LBBB)

Any Q-wave in leads V_2–V_3 ≥ 0.02 s or QS complex in leads V_2 and V_3

Q-wave ≥ 0.03 s and ≥ 0.1 mV deep or QS complex in leads I, II, aVL, aVF, or V_4–V_6 in any two leads of a contiguous lead grouping (I, aVL,V_6; V_4–V_6; II, III, and aVF)[a]

R-wave ≥ 0.04 s in V_1–V_2 and R/S ≥ 1 with a concordant positive T-wave in the absence of a conduction defect

---

[a]The same criteria are used for supplemental leads V_7–V_9, and for the Cabrera frontal plane lead grouping.

Table 4. ECG changes associated with prior myocardial infarction

---

False positives
  Benign early repolarization
  LBBB
  Pre-excitation
  Brugada syndrome
  Peri-/myocarditis
  Pulmonary embolism
  Subarachnoid haemorrhage
  Metabolic disturbances such as hyperkalaemia
  Failure to recognize normal limits for J-point displacement
  Lead transposition or use of modified Mason–Likar
    configuration[24]
  Cholecystitis
False negatives
  Prior myocardial infarction with Q-waves and/or persistent
    ST elevation
  Paced rhythm
  LBBB

Table 5. Common ECG pitfalls in diagnosing myocardial infarction

7. Management

Patients with an initial ECG reading that reveals new or presumably new ST segment depression and/or T wave inversion, although not considered candidates for fibrinolytic therapy, should be treated as though they are suffering from MI without ST elevation or unstable angina (a distinction to be made subsequently after scrutiny of serial ECGs and serum cardiac marker measurements). In patients with a clinical history suggestive of STEMI and an initial nondiagnostic ECG reading (i.e., no ST segment deviation or T wave inversion), serial tracings should be obtained while the patients are being evaluated in the emergency department.

Emergency department staff can be alerted to the sudden development of ST segment elevation by periodic visual inspection of the bedside ECG monitor, by continuous ST segment recording, or by auditory alarms when the ST segment deviation exceeds programmed limits. Decision aids such as computer-based diagnostic algorithms, identification of high-risk clinical indicators, rapid determination of cardiac serum markers, two-dimensional echocardiographic screening for regional wall motion abnormalities, and myocardial perfusion imaging have greatest clinical utility when the ECG reading is nondiagnostic. In an effort to improve the cost-effectiveness of care of patients with a chest pain syndrome, nondiagnostic ECG reading, and low suspicion of MI but in whom the diagnosis has not been entirely excluded, many medical centers have developed critical pathways that involve a coronary observation unit with a goal of ruling out MI in less than 12 hours.

Once the diagnosis of coronary artery disease is made, the management depends upon the severity of the underlying severity of the disease. The treating physician has to diagnose the clinical scenario appropriately as the treatment largely depends of the initial diagnosis. Stable coronary artery disease could be managed conservatively whereas acute coronary syndrome has to be managed very aggressively. Select patients have to be considered for early invasive strategy too.

The prehospital care of patients with suspected STEMI is a crucial element bearing directly on the likelihood of survival. Most deaths associated with STEMI occur within the first hour of its onset and are usually caused by ventricular fibrillation. Accordingly, the importance of the immediate implementation of definitive resuscitative efforts and of rapidly transporting the patient to a hospital cannot be overemphasized.

Major components of the delay from the onset of symptoms consistent with acute myocardial infarction (MI) to reperfusion include the following: (1) the time for the patient to recognize the seriousness of the problem and seek medical attention; (2) prehospital evaluation, treatment, and transportation; (3) the time for diagnostic measures and initiation of treatment in the hospital (e.g., "door-to-needle" time for patients receiving a thrombolytic agent and "door-to-balloon" time for patients undergoing a catheter-based reperfusion strategy); and (4) the time from initiation of treatment to restoration of flow (Figure 4). Thrombolytic therapy is vital for early reperfusion and this has been discussed in other chapters.

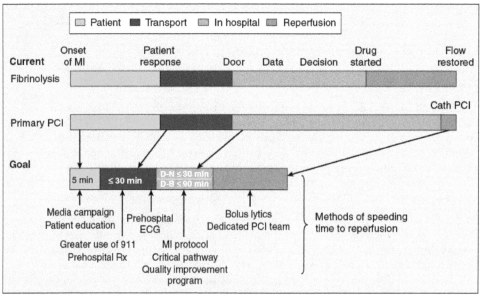

(Modified from Antman EM, Anbe DT, Armstrong PW, et al: ACC/AHA guidelines for the management of patients with ST-elevation myocardial infarction: A report of the American College of Cardiology/ American Heart Association Task Force on Practice Guidelines [Committee to Revise the 1999 Guidelines for the Management of Patients with Acute Myocardial Infarction]. Circulation 110:e82, 2004.)

Fig. 4.

Adjunctive medical therapy is a critical component of therapy for STEMI and confers benefit in addition to that gained by reperfusion therapies, regardless of method of reperfusion (Table 6).

Ancillary therapy can be used to facilitate and enhance coronary reperfusion or to limit the consequences of myocardial ischemia. Early, aggressive use of antiplatelet therapies, such as aspirin, and clopidogrel, confers significant additional mortality benefit when given as adjuncts to thrombolysis or PCI. Beta-blockers, angiotensin-converting enzyme inhibitors in appropriately selected patients, and 3-hydroxy-3-methylglutaryl CoA reductase inhibitors (statins) have all been shown to reduce the risk of cardiovascular events and mortality in patients who have STEMI. Therapies such as nitroglycerin and morphine have no mortality benefit but may improve symptoms and reduce ischemic burden. Calcium-channel blockers and prophylactic anti-arrhythmic drug therapy (lidocaine) may increase mortality. The suggested benefit of metabolic modulation at the myocyte level with electrolytes, glucose, and insulin seen in small, early trials has not been reproduced in larger, randomized studies.

Mechanisms and clinical effects of adjunctive therapies for patients who have ST elevation myocardial infarction

Agent	Mechanism	Clinical Effect
Adjunctive therapies for AMI		
Aspirin	Antiplatelet	Improve survival
		Decrease reinfarction, CVA
Thienopyridines (clopidogrel, ticlopidine)	Antiplatelet	Recommended in aspirin-allergic patients
		Decrease death, MI, CVA in NSTE ACS
Glycoprotein IIb/IIIa inhibitors	Antiplatelet	Decrease MI, ischemic complications following primary PCI
		Decrease death or MI in high-risk NSTE ACS
Unfractionated heparin	Antithrombin	Decrease death and MI in prefibrinolytic era
Low molecular weight heparins	Antithrombin	Reduce cardiac events in NSTE ACS versus unfractionated heparin
Direct thrombin inhibitors	Antithrombin	Recommended in heparin-induced thrombocytopenia
Beta-brockers	Decrease myocardial oxygen demand ($\downarrow$HR, $\downarrow$BP)	Improve survival
		Reduce infract size, ventricular arrhythmias, recurrent ischemia
Adjunctive therapies for AMI		
ACE Inhibitors	Vasodilator (BP)	Improve survival
	Prevent LV remodeling	Decrease heart failure, LV dysfunction
IV nitroglycerine	Venous, arterial, coronary vasodilator ($\downarrow$BP, $\downarrow$preload)	No effect on survival
		Decrease recurrent ischemia
HMG CoA Reductase Inhibitors	Lipid lowering	Decrease future CV death and MI
	Anti-inflammatory	May decrease early ischemic events
Magnesium	Myocardial protective	Therapy for torsades depointes
	Anti-arrhythmic	May improve reperfusion outcomes
Calcium-channel blocker	Decrease myocardial oxygen demand ($\downarrow$HR, $\downarrow$BP)	No survival benefit
		Possible use in beta-blocker–intolerant patients without CHF or LV dysfunction
Warfarin	Oral anticoagulant	Reduced embolic risk with atrial fibrilliation. LV thrombus or dysfunction
Glucose-insulin potassium infusion	Metabolic modulator	May improve intracellular myocardial energy stores and outcome

Abbreviations: ACS, acute coronary syndrome; BP, blood pressure; CHF, congestive heart failure; CV, cardiovascular; CVA, cerebrovascular accident; HR, heart rate; IV, intravenous; LV, left ventricular; MI, myocardial infarction; NSTE, non–ST-segment elevation; PCI, percutaneous coronary intervention.

Adapted from Sura AC. et al.

Table 6.

8. Conclusion

Although improvements in the management of patients who have STEMI have led to a decline in acute and long-term fatality rates, reperfusion and ancillary therapies remain underused. Several initiatives (eg. Get With the Guidelines in USA) are designed to improve adherence to guidelines and access to appropriate reperfusion therapies. To date, clinical advancement is judged on achieving and maintaining epicardial artery patency. New fibrinolytics and combination therapies will continue to evolve. There will be technological advances and improvement in operator skills for PCI. The ultimate goal for the management of STEMI remains unchanged: to open occluded arteries quickly in carefully screened patients and in a cost-effective manner.

9. References

[1] Rosamond W, Flegal K, Furie K, et al. Heart disease and stroke statistics--2008 update: a report from the American Heart Association Statistics Committee and Stroke Statistics Subcommittee. Circulation 2008; 117:e25.
[2] Lloyd-Jones D, Adams RJ, Brown TM, et al. Executive summary: heart disease and stroke statistics--2010 update: a report from the American Heart Association. Circulation 2010; 121:948.
[3] Towfighi A, Zheng L, Ovbiagele B. Sex-specific trends in midlife coronary heart disease risk and prevalence. Arch Intern Med 2009; 169:1762.
[4] Deedwania PC, Carbajal EV. Silent myocardial ischemia. A clinical perspective. Arch Intern Med 1991; 151:2373.
[5] Lopez AD, Mathers CD, Ezzati M, et al. Global and regional burden of disease and risk factors, 2001: systematic analysis of population health data. Lancet 2006; 367:1747.
[6] Yusuf S, Reddy S, Ounpuu S, Anand S. Global burden of cardiovascular diseases: part I: general considerations, the epidemiologic transition, risk factors, and impact of urbanization. Circulation 2001; 104:2746.
[7] Goyal A, Yusuf S. The burden of cardiovascular disease in the Indian subcontinent. Indian J Med Res 2006; 124:235.
[8] Critchley J, Liu J, Zhao D, et al. Explaining the increase in coronary heart disease mortality in Beijing between 1984 and 1999. Circulation 2004; 110:1236.
[9] Rodríguez T, Malvezzi M, Chatenoud L, et al. Trends in mortality from coronary heart and cerebrovascular diseases in the Americas: 1970-2000. Heart 2006; 92:453.
[10] Beaglehole R, Reddy S, Leeder SR. Poverty and human development: the global implications of cardiovascular disease. Circulation 2007; 116:1871.
[11] Kloner RA, Jennings RB: Consequences of brief ischemia: Stunning, preconditioning, and their clinical implications: Part 1. *Circulation* 2001; 104:2981.
[12] Downey JM, Cohen MV: Reducing infarct size in the setting of acute myocardial infarction. *Prog Cardiovasc Dis* 2006; 48:363.
[13] Alpert JS, Thygesen K, Antman E, Bassand JP. Myocardial infarction redefined--a consensus document of The Joint European Society of Cardiology/American College of Cardiology Committee for the redefinition of myocardial infarction. J Am Coll Cardiol 2000; 36:959.
[14] Thygesen K, Alpert JS, White HD, Joint ESC/ACCF/AHA/WHF Task Force for the Redefinition of Myocardial Infarction. Universal definition of myocardial infarction. Eur Heart J 2007; 28:2525.

Part 2

Diagnostics of Ischemic Heart Disease

2

Inflammatory Biomarkers in Ischemic Heart Disease

Mette Bjerre

The Medical Research Laboratories, Institute of Clinical Medicine,
Faculty of Health Sciences, Aarhus University
Denmark

1. Introduction

Ischemic heart disease (IHD) is one of the main groups within the class of cardiovascular diseases (CVD), and IHD is the most common single cause of morbidity and mortality in the Western world (Gaziano et al., 2006). According to the American Heart Association Statistics Committee one in three individuals has one or more forms of CVD (Rosamond et al., 2007).

The importance of inflammation in the pathogenesis of IHD, such as, acute myocardial infarct (AMI) and coronary artery disease (CAD), has long been established. A large body of evidence suggests that inflammation plays a key role in CVD, however, the mechanisms in the various stages of the pathological process is not completely understood (Carden and Granger, 2000). Inflammation is a complex of defensive mechanisms reacting to the entry of harmful agents into the organism or cells, in order to eliminate or repair damaged cells or tissue and to restore homeostasis. This broad definition indicates that inflammation does not only accompany infectious diseases, but also other conditions causing cell, tissue or organ damage.

The identified risk factors for IHD include both lifestyle and biological factors, such as smoking, high blood pressure, high cholesterol levels, obesity, and diabetes that all appear to exaggerate many of the vascular alterations elicited by ischemia and reperfusion. Diabetes and CVD often appear as two sides of a coin: on one side, diabetes has been rated as an equivalent of CVD, and conversely, many patients with established CVD suffer from overt or incipient diabetes (Ryden et al., 2007). The mortality from AMI is almost increased five-fold in diabetic patients compared with non-diabetics (Hansen et al., 2007) and diabetes and low-grade inflammation is closely related (Flyvbjerg, 2010). Obesity is seen at epidemic proportions all over the world, and is a significant risk factor for, and contributing factor to increased morbidity and mortality, most importantly from CVD and diabetes (Lavie et al., 2009a). Likewise, obesity is also associated with low-grade inflammation and CVD (Yudkin et al., 1999; Bastard et al., 2006).

Although the combination of traditional risk factors such as age, gender, lifestyle, dyslipidemia, hypertension and diabetes are well established for the prediction of cardiovascular mortality (e.g. the Framingham coronary risk score), these algorithms do not adequately differentiate individuals at moderate risk. Indeed, not all patients with CVD will have conventional risk factors and not all patients with risk factors will develop CVD (Khot et al., 2003). Both biomarkers of early disease and plaque instability have therefore been sought, and the development of new markers to diagnose and prevent CVD is an important public health goal worldwide. However, a recent report showed that the addition of a multi-marker score including 10 new markers to conventional risk factors added only a moderate increase in the ability to grade the risk in the general population (Wang et al., 2006).

Several inflammatory biomarkers have been shown to represent important cardiovascular risk factors, and this review will primarily focus on the complement system, the acute-phase reactant C-reactive protein (CRP), and the antimicrobial peptides: α-defensins. Whether these inflammatory proteins mediate IHD themselves or solely serve as markers of systemic inflammation and cardiovascular risk stratification is still intensely studied.

2. Inflammation and IHD

Growing evidence indicates that IHD is a broad syndrome with multiple pathogenetic and aetiological components, which may not be the same in all patients. Extensive literature supports the role of inflammation in IHD (Mehta and Li, 1999; Ross, 1999). Inflammatory cells, inflammatory proteins and inflammatory responses from vascular cells are all reported to play crucial roles in various stages of a number of CVD (Carden and Granger, 2000). Some of the inflammatory mechanisms of IHD include, among others, endothelial dysfunction, oxidative stress and vascular calcification, that all seems to play an important role for the development of cardiovascular disease.

Although timely restoration of blood-flow after a myocardial ischemic event is essential to prevent irreversible cellular injury, it is widely recognized that the outcome of tissue injury not only depends on the duration of the ischemic event, but also on reperfusion as a critical factor (Khalil et al., 2006). Paradoxically, the reperfusion exacerbates severe tissue damage, especially after longer periods of ischemia. The intensity of the inflammatory reaction in post-ischemic tissue can be so strong that the injury response to reperfusion can be manifested in distant organs (Carden and Granger, 2000).

The ischemia-reperfusion injury (IRI) results in a local and systemic inflammatory response characterized by the production of reactive oxygen species (ROS), leucocyte-endothelial cell adhesion, complement activation, endothelial leucocyte migration, increased micro-vascular permeability and decreased endothelial-dependent relaxation (Carden and Granger, 2000). Within minutes of reperfusion ROS are generated (Cannon, 2005), stimulating the release of cytokines and expression of adhesion molecules on damaged cells in reperfused tissue. Several hours after onset of reperfusion, neutrophils and other inflammatory cells are activated (Frangogiannis et al., 2002; Frangogiannis, 2007) and adhere to the damaged cell membranes (Zimmerman et al., 1990; Vinten-Johansen, 2004) for further enhancement of the inflammatory response. Thus, IRI poses major problems in the clinic, and effective therapies are required.

3. Inflammatory biomarkers

Recent research has been focused on identifying biomarkers, which alone or in combination with other risk markers could be useful in monitoring the treatment and as prognostic markers for future coronary syndromes and cardiac death in patients with IHD.

In 2001, a National Institute of Health working group defined a biomarker as "a characteristic that is objectively measured and evaluated as an indicator of normal biological processes, pathogenic processes or pharmacological responses to a therapeutic intervention (BiomarkersDefinitionsWorkingGroup, 2001). Biomarkers are traditionally specific proteins circulating in the body fluids that become altered as a consequence of disease progression or the effect of a therapeutic intervention and can be divided into different categories:

- Disease-predictive
- Diagnostic
- Prognostic
- Disease-associated
- Therapeutic efficacy.

A number of inflammatory biomarkers have been associated with cardiovascular diseases. Biomarker measurements can help explain empirical results of clinical trials by relating the effects of interventions on molecular and cellular pathways to clinical responses, thus providing an opportunity for researchers to gain a mechanistic understanding.

3.1 The complement system

The complement system is an innate, cytotoxic host defence that normally functions to eliminate pathogens and facilitates the clearance of damaged tissue and apoptotic cells. However, excessive activation of the system may lead to uncontrolled tissue damage. The relevance of complement activation in myocardial ischemia was already proposed more than four decades ago (Hill and Ward, 1971). The inflammatory mechanisms by which tissue injury after an AMI occurs has not been fully elucidated, but strong evidence obtained from animal models, as well as clinical studies, support the hypothesis of a role for the complement system in IHD (Bjerre et al., 2008).

The complement system is a biochemical cascade, which helps clear pathogens from an organism, and is thus one part of a larger immune system. Three pathways of complement activation have been identified (Figure 1), known as the classical, the alternative and the lectin pathway. The classical pathway is initiated by C1q binding to antibody complexes (Cooper, 1985) whereas the alternative pathway is initiated by spontaneous and direct activation of C3 (Muller-Eberhard, 1988). The lectin pathway is initiated either through ficolin (M-, L- or H-ficolin) (Matsushita et al., 2001; Frederiksen et al., 2005), by pattern recognition of N-acetyl-glucosamine-rich polysaccharides or through mannan-binding lectin (MBL) binding to certain carbohydrate structures (Ikeda et al., 1987; Thiel et al., 1997; Holmskov et al., 2003).

Activation of the complement system promotes three main biological activities (Walport, 2001): I) recruitment of inflammatory cells by anaphylatoxins (C3a, C4a, and C5a), leading to accumulation of activated polymorph nuclear leukocytes directly involved in tissue destruction, II) opsonisation of pathogens for phagocytosis by the generation of C3b, and III) lysis of the pathogen by the generation of a membrane attack complex (MAC, C5b-9) penetrating the cell membrane. The loss of membrane integrity destroys the ability to control the concentration of salt within the cell and the cell is killed due to this osmotic instability. MAC formed in the absence of target membranes binds to S-protein, which inhibits the membrane-damaging effect, and creates a stable non-lytic soluble C5b-9 form (sMAC, sC5b-9) (Fosbrink et al., 2005).

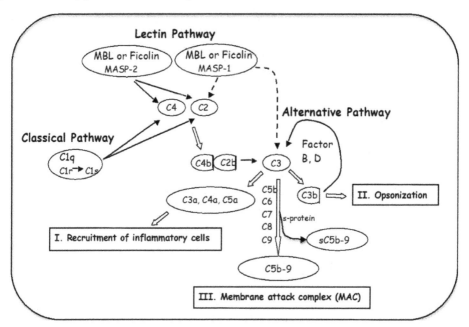

Fig. 1. The complement system can be activated through three pathways, which merge at the cleavage of C3, leading to the effector mechanisms: **I.** recruitment of inflammatory cells, **II.** opsonisation and **III.** the generation of the membrane attack complex (MAC, C5b-9) for cell lysis.

3.1.1 Role of complement in endothelial function

Ischemia and reperfusion are potent activators of the complement system and both clinical and experimental studies in different organs have shown local deposition of complement (Riedemann and Ward, 2003; Arumugam et al., 2004). It has traditionally been assumed that the liver is the source of complement proteins that participate in these events, but complement proteins are produced in several organs of the body, including the heart and the endothelium.

The human heart expresses mRNAs, translated into proteins, for all of the components of the classical complement pathway (Yasojima et al., 1998b). This production is up-regulated in areas of myocardial infarct, and the classical complement pathway was found to be fully activated on injured myocardial tissue. In addition, production of C3 and C9 mRNAs and their protein products was significantly increased in isolated rabbit heart after reperfusion injury, and the production by heart in this circumstance substantially exceeds that of the normal liver (Yasojima et al., 1998a).

Endothelial cells also represent one of the extrahepatic sources of complement components and regulators. Due to the strategic position along the surface of the vessel wall, they may supply both the circulating blood and the extravascular fluids with these proteins. Most of the information on the production of complement components by endothelial cells has been obtained using human umbilical vein endothelial cells (HUVECs). HUVECs cultured in serum free media were reported to synthesize functional C3, C5, C6, C8, and C9 and assembling of the MAC complex was found, indicating that C7 was produced as well (Johnson and Hetland, 1991). The C7 production was later confirmed (Langeggen et al., 2000) and a small production of C5, C6, C8, and C9 demonstrated by RT-PCR and Northern blot was reported (Langeggen et al., 2001). Activation of the complement cascade leads to the formation of the C5b-9 complex on the cell surface that can cause cell death. However, when the numbers of C5b-9 molecules are limited on host cell membranes, it can activate signalling pathways leading to cell cycle activation and cell survival (Niculescu and Rus, 2001).

The reduction in the capacity of the endothelium to maintain the homeostasis leads to the development of pathological inflammatory processes and vascular diseases. An intact endothelium is a fully biocompatible surface that is not recognized by the complement system. However, blood contact with a damaged endothelium will lead to a certain degree of activation of the defence system. Complement activation results in the formation of several biological active components including C3a, C5a, iC3b, and C5b-9. In addition, to stimulate inflammatory response C5a have been reported to induce production of chemokines and cytokines (Czermak et al., 1999).

3.1.2 Mechanism of complement in IHD

Cardiovascular risk factors (e.g., hypercholesterolemia, hypertension, smoking, diabetes, stress) cause oxidative stress that alters the endothelial cell capacity (Esper et al., 2006; Kyrou and Tsigos, 2007), and thus dysfunction of the endothelium has been implicated in the pathophysiology of different forms of CVD (reviewed by (Endemann and Schiffrin, 2004)). Human endothelial cells have been shown to generate reactive oxygen intermediates in response to hyperglycaemia and lead to dysfunction in type 2 diabetic patients (Bellin et al., 2006). Endothelial dysfunction has been shown to have a prognostic value in patients with chest pain (Neunteufl et al., 2000) and both C-reactive protein (CRP) and C3a were found to be elevated in patients with unstable angina pectoris (Kostner et al., 2006). Elevated plasma levels of C3 was independently associated with MI after accounting for traditional cardiovascular risk factors and CRP in patients with MI, whereas the association of CRP was dependent of C3 (Carter et al., 2009).

A number of *in vitro* studies using HUVECs have shown that under anoxic conditions the endothelial cells become activators of the complement system. Collard and co-workers showed increased MBL, C3, and iC3b deposition after hypoxia/reoxygenation (Collard et al., 2000; Collard et al., 2001). MBL deposition was attenuated in the presence of MBL ligands indicating the presence of MBL neo-epitopes on the surface of the endothelial cells. Apoptotic endothelial cells deposited C1 and C3d, thus activating the complement system (Mold and Morris, 2001). Experimental studies in porcine and rabbits reported that complement activation attenuates endothelium-dependent relaxation (Stahl et al., 1995; Lennon et al., 1996). The role of complement was mediated by the formation of C5b-9, but not through the generation of the anaphylatoxin C3a and C5a.

Hill et al. were the first to report a role for the complement system after an ischemic event in a rat model of AMI (Hill and Ward, 1971). The association between AMI and complement activation was later confirmed in baboons showing deposition of complement factors in the infarcted tissue (Pinckard et al., 1980; McManus et al., 1983). Later, several studies of experimental myocardial I/R showed deposition of complement; C1 (Vakeva et al., 1994), MBL and C3 (Walsh et al., 2005), C4, C5 (McManus et al., 1983; Crawford et al., 1988), C6 (Ito et al., 1996), and C5b-9 (Vakeva et al., 1994). MBL knock-out (KO) mice were protected from heart I/R injury, but when reconstituted with human recombinant MBL, I/R injury similar to that in wild type mice was found. Mice deficient in C2 and factor B (C2/B KO) were also protected form heart I/R injury but no protection was found in C1q or factor D KO mice (Walsh et al., 2005). In a murine model of coronary artery ischemia the involvement of natural IgM antibodies has been linked to both the classical and the lectin pathways (Zhang et al., 2006a; Zhang et al., 2006b). Mice bearing an altered natural IgM repertoire were significantly protected based on the reduced infarct size, limited apoptosis of cardiomyocytes, and decreased neutrophil infiltration.

In addition to direct lytic activity, C5b-9 also directly attenuates endothelium-dependent (i.e., NO-mediated) relaxation (Stahl et al., 1995). Furthermore, C5b-9 is found to play a role in leucocyte activation, adherence and chemotaxis by induction of different cytokines (Kilgore et al., 1996; Vakeva et al., 1998). Also, activation of endothelial NF-kB and the stimulation of expression of endothelial adhesion molecules have been observed. Furthermore, a role for C5b-9 in mediating myocardial apoptosis after ischemia-reperfusion was demonstrated in a model of rat myocardial IRI (Vakeva et al., 1998). We have shown that increased complement activity as indicated by MBL and sC5b-9 levels, was associated with increased risk of cardiac dysfunction in STEMI patients treated with pPCI (Haahr-Pedersen et al., 2009). High plasma MBL and low plasma sC5b-9 was independently associated with increased risk of cardiac dysfunction, likely due to increased complement activity during the ischemic and reperfusion process. The predictive value of low peripheral plasma sC5b-9 may be explained by an accumulation and activation of sC5b-9 in the infarcted myocardium. Furthermore, an elevated plasma sC5b-9 level was found in patients with chronic heart failure due to IHD (Bjerre et al., 2010). In addition, an independent association between sC5b-9, insulin resistance and endothelial dysfunction was found, which may suggest that insulin resistance leading to endothelial activation results in activation of the complement system thus damaging the heart.

3.1.3 Therapeutic inhibition of complement in IHD

Based on the studies discussed above, regulation of the complement system seems to be of great importance. Indeed, several animal studies point to a possible beneficial role of complement depletion in the treatment of post-ischemic MI; reviewed by (Bjerre et al., 2008; Diepenhorst et al., 2009). Unfortunately, clinical studies focused on complement depletion in humans, especially the use of anti-C5 antibodies, primarily Pexelizumab, have largely been disappointing and not proven effective in the setting of CVD, discussed in details elsewhere: (Bjerre et al., 2008; Diepenhorst et al., 2009; Banz and Rieben, 2011).

Although much of the preclinical work and data accumulated in the past years have been positive, the problem with complement-mediated damage in IR-injury was not "easy to fix". Thus conclusions drawn from animal studies should be extrapolated to the human settings with caution. It may lie in the fact that complement activation represents only a part of the cascade of attack directed against the vasculature. An exaggerated blockade of the immune system may increase the susceptibility to infections, thus a well-balanced inhibition of the complement activation is required in order to avoid side effects of pharmaceutically induced modification of the immune system. Direct targeting may be the key to future treatment strategies, including targeting of the complement inhibitor to the site of injury by localized intravascular application.

3.2 C-reactive protein

C-reactive protein (CRP), an acute-phase reactant mainly produced by hepatocytes in response to interleukin (IL) 6, is a nonspecific marker of systemic inflammation, and is the most intensively studied inflammatory biomarker in CVD. In addition, a large number of reports have shown that CRP may be implicated in the pathogenesis of many chronic diseases, including diabetes, cancer and alzheimer dementia, and major CVDs, such as, coronary heart disease (CHD), AMI and IHD (Clyne and Olshaker, 1999; Hirschfield and Pepys, 2003; Lavie et al., 2009b). Of note, CRP levels has been associated with the size of the infarct (de Beer et al., 1982).

The concentration of CRP increases rapidly; it may raise hundreds-fold after acute tissue injury or inflammation, and declines rapidly with resolution of the injurious process. In healthy persons, normal CRP levels are generally considered to be < 3 mg/L (Shine et al., 1981).

3.2.1 High sensitive CRP and IHD

In the 1990s, rapid and more precise methods of quantifying CRP was established and CRP levels measured as low as 0.04 mg/L were possible, referred to as high sensitive (hs) CRP (Jaye and Waites, 1997). Low-grade inflammation is found in IHD, and CRP levels are not as increased as compared to other inflammatory conditions. Therefore, a cardiovascular risk scale according to hsCRP levels is recommended by the American Heart Association and Centers for Disease Control and Prevention (Pearson et al., 2003).

Individuals with hsCRP levels;

- <1 mg/L are at lower relative risk for cardiovascular events,
- 1 to 3 mg/L are at intermediate risk,
- >3 mg/L are at higher relative risk.

In the Copenhagen City Heart study, investigating more than 10,000 apparently healthy participants, elevated hsCRP levels were found to be associated with increased risk of IHD. In fact, the risk of IHD was more than doubled (HR=2.2, 1.6-2.9) in individuals with CRP levels above 3 mg/L as compared to individuals with CRP levels below 1 mg/L (Zacho et al., 2008).

3.2.2 Possible links between hsCRP and IHD

Inflammation clearly plays a clinically significant role in the development of CVD. Consequently, as a marker of inflammation, hsCRP has been studied extensively in patients with CVD. The predictive value of hsCRP has been widely investigated but the results are contradictive. More than 20 large prospective trials have shown that hsCRP is an independent predictor of future cardiovascular events (Ridker, 2007). In the most recent comprehensive meta-analysis studies of cardiovascular risk factors (more than 50 prospective studies with over 160,000 participants, none of them with a history of coronary heart disease or stroke) (Kaptoge et al., 2010), hsCRP was consistently found to be an independent predictor of CVD. However, the association with ischemic vascular disease depends considerably on conventional risk factors and other markers of inflammation. A critical review by Levinson and colleagues argues that hsCRP is poor discrimination over a wide range of values when used in conjunction with risk factors for lipoprotein lipids, hypertension, metabolic syndrome, and diabetes (Levinson et al., 2004). Danesh and colleagues published a study, performed in a high-risk population with nonfatal myocardial infarct, which questioned the role of CRP in the assessment of cardiovascular risk. However, hsCRP maintained a predictive value after adjustments for smoking and hypertension (Danesh et al., 2004).

A panel of multiple biomarkers, 10 biomarkers in total including hsCRP, was used for prediction of death and major cardiovascular event in more than 3000 participants of the Framingham Off-spring study followed for 10 years (Wang et al., 2006). As a single marker, hsCRP predicted risk of death but no major cardiovascular events after adjusting for other biomarkers, and individuals with high multimarker scores had almost 4 times as great a risk of death. Nonetheless, the authors concluded that the use of contemporary biomarkers adds only moderately to standard risk factors. In the Women's Health Study, CRP was found to be additive to LDL-cholesterol in predicting future CVD in healthy American women (n=28,263 apparently healthy postmenopausal women) (Ridker et al., 2000a). Of the 12 markers measured (including hsCRP and IL-6), hs-CRP was the strongest uni-variant predictor of cardiovascular events, and the only plasma marker predicting risk after adjustment in a multi-variant analysis. This was confirmed in a large meta-analysis of hsCRP as a single biomarker in patients with stable CAD, but the authors concluded that a routine measurement of CRP should not be recommended as a single prognostic biomarker (Hemingway et al., 2010). However, in combination with other biomarkers, hsCRP seems to add significant information to traditional risk factors for CVD, and the value of adding hsCRP to standard risk equations was noted in separate cohorts of asymptomatic (middle-aged or elderly) men and women (Lavie et al., 2009b).

In the Caerphilly Prospective Heart Disease Study, Mendall and colleagues, showed a significant and positive association between CRP and incidents of IHD, not affected by ischemia history (Mendall et al., 2000). However, after adjustment of lifestyle risk factors (such as smoking and obesity) only the association with all-cause mortality remained significant. Plasma hsCRP was not found as an independent predictor of long-term IHD risk in a 13-year-follow-up study of men with no previous history of IHD (n=1982) (St-Pierre et al., 2005). The authors thus concluded that neither CRP nor the systemic inflammation appeared to have a direct role in the development of IHD. But the association of hsCRP with IHD may be that CRP levels are raised non-specifically by a variety of exposures that are themselves implicated in the pathogenesis of IHD (Figure 2).

A connection between CRP and activation of the complement system was proposed more than 35 years ago, after the discovery of aggregated or ligand-complexed human CRP was able to bind to C1q and activate the classical pathway (Kaplan and Volanakis, 1974; Siegel et al., 1974; Jiang et al., 1991), thus mediating the functions summarized in Figure 1. CRP was later found to co-localize with activated complement fragments in atherosclerotic lesions (Bhakdi et al., 1999; Yasojima et al., 2001) and CRP-mediated complement activation in the arterial wall may be considered as an important pathogenic feature in CVD.

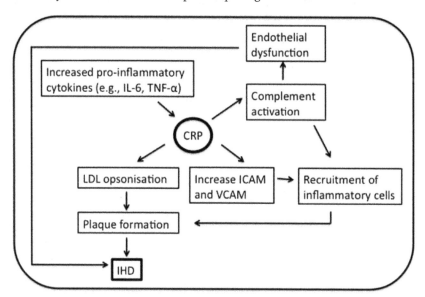

Fig. 2. Schematic depiction of potential mechanisms of CRP involvement in the pathogenesis of IHD.

A number of pro-inflammatory cytokines have been shown to play roles in the process leading to IHD, but IL-6, in particular, appears to have a central role, e.g. by stimulating the liver to increase the CRP production. However, even with a strong correlation between IL-6 and CRP, IL-6 was found to predict future AMI in a group of apparently healthy men (Ridker et al., 2000b).

CRP binds to apolipoprotein-containing lipoproteins like LDL (de Beer et al., 1982) and very low-density lipoprotein (VLDL) (Rowe et al., 1984), which may be of considerable importance in the pathogenesis of CVD. More recent studies revealed that CRP preferentially binds to modified forms of LDL; enzymatically modified LDL (Bhakdi et al., 1999) and oxidized LDL (Chang et al., 2002), and CRP was reported to mediate LDL uptake by macrophages (Zwaka et al., 2001). Opsonisation of LDL lead to monocyte infiltration and the formation of foam cells resulting in plaque formation and eventually IHD.

CRP was found to cause expression of cell adhesion molecules with a significant dose-dependent expression of ICAM-1, VCAM-1 and E-selectin in human umbilical vein endothelial cells (HUVEC) following CRP stimulation (Pasceri et al., 2000). Furthermore, production of chemokines monocyte chemoattractant protein-1 (MCP-1), which plays an important role in recruitment of monocytes into the vessel wall and thus the formation of plaques, was directly induced by CRP (Pasceri et al., 2001).

3.2.3 Is CRP a potential therapeutic in prevention of IHD?

As described in the previous section, CRP is reported to be associated with a wide range of biomarkers and risk factors of IHD. Thus, overestimating of the true effect of hsCRP on CVD risk, because of confounding effects, constitute a challenge. Support for a role of CRP in the pathogenesis of CVD comes primary from epidemiologic studies, which in general have observed an association between elevated plasma CRP and cardiovascular events.

Although hsCRP may not be the ideal marker of IHD, it seems to be very reliable, and hsCRP is a simple, non-invasive, commercially available, inexpensive and reproducible biomarker. CRP measurement has a lot of advantages; the protein is stable and the concentration is not subjected to time-of-the day variations (Meier-Ewert et al., 2001). Thus, determination of baseline hsCRP for cardiovascular risk prediction may be performed without concern for diurnal variation.

Availability of drugs to block CRP binding and its effects *in vivo* would provide a powerful tool for determining whether CRP is just a marker or does indeed participate in the pathogenesis of CVD complications. Griselli and colleagues (Griselli et al., 1999) showed that injection of human CRP in a rat model of AMI enhanced the infarct size, of note rat CRP does not activate rat complement, whereas human CRP activate both rat and human complement. However, in vivo complement depletion, by cobra venom factor, completely abrogated this. A similar effect was later found by administration of a specific synthetic CRP-inhibitor, 1,6-bis(phosphocholine)-hexane, which reduced the infarct size and thus provided promising results for therapeutic inhibition of CRP (Pepys et al., 2006).

Statins lower the levels of LDL-cholesterol and CRP. Ridker and colleagues showed, in a sub-population (n= 3745) derived from the Pravastatin or Atorvastatin Evaluation and Infection Therapy–Thrombolysis in Myocardial Infarction 22 (PROVE IT–TIMI 22) study, that patients with low hsCRP levels after statin treatment had improved cardiovascular outcome (Ridker et al., 2005). Patients in whom statin therapy resulted in hsCRP levels below 2 mg/L overall had better clinical outcomes regardless of the LDL-cholesterol level achieved. Recently, a study JUPITER: Justification for the Use of Statins in Prevention: an Intervention Trial Evaluating Rosuvastatin (n=17802), of healthy individuals without history of CVD but hsCRP > 2 mg/L and low LDL concentration, showed beneficial effect of Rosuvastatin (Ridker et al., 2007; Kones, 2010; Ridker et al., 2010). The study was terminated due to a great risk-reduction in AMI, CVD and death from cardiovascular causes, indicating that part of the statin effect may be mediated through lowering CRP.

Aside from whether measurement of CRP is useful in assessments of CVD, studies are needed to help determine if CRP is a mediator or a marker of CVD. Zacho et al. showed that genetic variants that are associated with a lifelong increased plasma CRP level are not associated with increased risk of IHD (Zacho et al., 2008), indicating CRP as a marker but not as an actual contributor.

3.3 Anti-microbial peptides

The involvement of polymorphonuclear neutrophils (PMNs) in the pathogenesis of CVD has received relatively little attention, despite their presence in the atherosclerotic plaques (Quinn et al., 2008). PMN counts have been reported as independent risk factors for cardiovascular outcome (Madjid et al., 2004) and during inflammation PMNs are activated in order to enhance the inflammatory response and releases antimicrobial peptides into circulation.

Anti-microbial peptides are polypeptides of fewer than 100 amino acids. The human innate immune system includes two main families; defensins and cathelicidins. Defensins, also termed human neutrophil peptides (HNP) as they are found in large amounts in neutrophils, are secreted during phagocytosis as a first line of defence against invading organisms (Ganz, 2003).

3.3.1 α-defensins

Three different classes of defensin are identified in mammals, two of which are found in humans; α- and β-defensin (Ganz, 1987). The human family of α-defensins are composed of 3 closely related gene products, also referred to as human neutrophil peptides 1-3 (HNPs-1-3) and HNP4, HNP5 and HNP6. The α-defensins are cationic peptides, cysteine-rich peptides of approximately 3 kDa and are normally sequestered in the granules of neutrophils, where they constitute 5% of the total cellular protein and are involved in the intracellular killing of prokaryotic organisms (Ganz, 1987). Under normal conditions, only small amounts of α-defensins (nanomolar range) are found in plasma. However, during inflammatory reactions, α-defensins are released extracellularly, which could exert harmful effects on host cells. Increased plasma concentrations of α-defensins have been described in several inflammatory diseases (Ganz, 2003; Klotman and Chang, 2006; de Leeuw and Lu, 2007).

3.3.2 Possible link between α-defensins and IHD

The cationic nature of the α-defensins prefers the negatively charged phospholipids of the bacterial membrane as target and avoids the more neutral charged mammalian cell membrane. However, both a direct and an indirect chemoattracting role of α-defensins has been reported for a number of cells (Oppenheim et al., 2003). In addition, α-defensin was found to promote oxidative stress and induces endothelial dysfunction by reducing the endothelium-dependent relaxation in porcine coronary arteries (Kougias et al., 2006). This effect is associated with increased superoxide radical production and decreased eNOS expression. Also, α-defensins is capable of forming complexes with C1q and MBL, thus playing a role in the regulation of both the classical and the lectin pathway of complement activation (Groeneveld et al., 2007).

Localization of α-defensins were analysed by the use of immunohistochemical staining of coronary arteries from patients with severe CVD or normal donor heart tissue (Barnathan et al., 1997). Of interest, α-defensin was found most prominently in association with intima smooth muscle cells of both normal or atherosclerotic vessels. α-defensins has been reported as an atherogenic agent by enhancing and promoting stable complexes with LDL particles, thus stimulating the binding to endothelial and smooth muscle cells (Higazi et al., 1997). In addition, in human cerebral vessels obtained during autopsy, α-defensin and LDL co-localized primary within the atherosclerotic areas, and the staining intensity correlated with the severity of the disease. The authors hypothesize that the small α-defensins may rapidly cross the endothelial barrier and gain access to sub-endothelial matrix and affording the binding of LDL and a complex relative resistant to degradation. Retention of LDL in the arteries may predispose to pro-atherogenic modifications, such as, oxidation and internalization by foam cells. In addition, an independent negative relationship between high-density lipoprotein (HDL) has later been described (Saraheimo et al., 2008). Furthermore, α-defensins were found to inhibit the fibrionolytic activity by binding to tissue plasminogen activator molecule (Kougias et al., 2005). In a small study of patients undergoing elective coronary artery catheterization, an accumulation of α-defensin in the human skin was described and the accumulated amount correlated with the severity of coronary artery disease (Nassar et al., 2007). Of note, no correlation between CRP and α-defensin was found in this study.

Chronic low-grade inflammation is a hallmark of obesity and diabetes, and has been causally linked to the development of premature CVD. In a group of type-1 diabetic patients, with a 10-year-follow-up-period of cardiovascular end-points, elevated baseline plasma α-defensin levels were an independent predictor for cardiovascular morbidity and mortality (Joseph et al., 2008). In a recent study, the risk of cardiovascular mortality was significantly increased with elevated plasma α-defensin levels in patients admitted for elective lower extremity artery surgery (Urbonaviciene et al., 2011). Surprisingly, patients with high α-defensin levels combined with high hs-CRP levels had a five time increased risk of cardiovascular death compared to patients in whom only one or none of the peptides was elevated.

4. Perspectives

Inflammatory biomarkers may have prognostic value for future cardiovascular risk stratification among individuals with high risk or a history of IHD, but they may also in particular be useful in apparently healthy individuals who might be at higher risk than estimated by the traditional risk factor scores. Using a biomarker profile that covers various aspects of the complex pathophysiology of IHD may increase the rational basis for cardiovascular risk assessment. As decribed above, a multiple inflammatory role of the combination of complement activation, CRP, LDL and α-defensins may participate in the pathogenesis of IHD and other CVD.

With the emergence of novel biomarkers for inflammation and vascular damage it may be possible to characterize different contributions of each of these major mechanisms to short- and long-term prognosis following CVD. Hopefully, patients may benefit from different therapeutic strategies depending on their personal biomarker profile in the future. So far, however, results about which biomarkers are the most suitable for diagnosis or prognosis of IHD remain conflicting, and further research within this field is needed.

5. References

Arumugam, T.V., Shiels, I.A., Woodruff, T.M., Granger, D.N. and Taylor, S.M. (2004) The role of the complement system in ischemia-reperfusion injury. Shock 21, 401-9.

Banz, Y. and Rieben, R. (2011) Role of complement and perspectives for intervention in ischemia-reperfusion damage. Ann Med.

Barnathan, E.S., Raghunath, P.N., Tomaszewski, J.E., Ganz, T., Cines, D.B. and Higazi, A.a.-R. (1997) Immunohistochemical localization of defensin in human coronary vessels. Am J Pathol 150, 1009-20.

Bastard, J.P., Maachi, M., Lagathu, C., Kim, M.J., Caron, M., Vidal, H., Capeau, J. and Feve, B. (2006) Recent advances in the relationship between obesity, inflammation, and insulin resistance. Eur Cytokine Netw 17, 4-12.

Bellin, C., de Wiza, D.H., Wiernsperger, N.F. and Rosen, P. (2006) Generation of reactive oxygen species by endothelial and smooth muscle cells: influence of hyperglycemia and metformin. Horm Metab Res 38, 732-9.

Bhakdi, S., Torzewski, M., Klouche, M. and Hemmes, M. (1999) Complement and atherogenesis: binding of CRP to degraded, nonoxidized LDL enhances complement activation. Arterioscler Thromb Vasc Biol 19, 2348-54.

BiomarkersDefinitionsWorkingGroup. (2001) Biomarkers and surrogate endpoints: preferred definitions and conceptual framework. Clin Pharmacol Ther 69, 89-95.

Bjerre, M., Hansen, T.K. and Flyvbjerg, A. (2008) Complement activation and cardiovascular disease. Horm Metab Res 40, 626-34.

Bjerre, M., Kistorp, C., Hansen, T.K., Faber, J., Lip, G.Y., Hildebrandt, P. and Flyvbjerg, A. (2010) Complement activation, endothelial dysfunction, insulin resistance and chronic heart failure. Scand Cardiovasc J 44, 260-6.

Cannon, R.O., 3rd. (2005) Mechanisms, management and future directions for reperfusion injury after acute myocardial infarction. Nat Clin Pract Cardiovasc Med 2, 88-94.

Carden, D.L. and Granger, D.N. (2000) Pathophysiology of ischaemia-reperfusion injury. J Pathol 190, 255-66.

Carter, A.M., Prasad, U.K. and Grant, P.J. (2009) Complement C3 and C-reactive protein in male survivors of myocardial infarction. Atherosclerosis 203, 538-43.

Chang, M.K., Binder, C.J., Torzewski, M. and Witztum, J.L. (2002) C-reactive protein binds to both oxidized LDL and apoptotic cells through recognition of a common ligand: Phosphorylcholine of oxidized phospholipids. Proc Natl Acad Sci U S A 99, 13043-8.

Clyne, B. and Olshaker, J.S. (1999) The C-reactive protein. J Emerg Med 17, 1019-25.

Collard, C.D., Montalto, M.C., Reenstra, W.R., Buras, J.A. and Stahl, G.L. (2001) Endothelial oxidative stress activates the lectin complement pathway: role of cytokeratin 1. Am J Pathol 159, 1045-54.

Collard, C.D., Vakeva, A., Morrissey, M.A., Agah, A., Rollins, S.A., Reenstra, W.R., Buras, J.A., Meri, S. and Stahl, G.L. (2000) Complement activation after oxidative stress: role of the lectin complement pathway. Am J Pathol 156, 1549-56.

Cooper, N.R. (1985) The classical complement pathway: activation and regulation of the first complement component. Adv Immunol 37, 151-216.

Crawford, M.H., Grover, F.L., Kolb, W.P., McMahan, C.A., O'Rourke, R.A., McManus, L.M. and Pinckard, R.N. (1988) Complement and neutrophil activation in the pathogenesis of ischemic myocardial injury. Circulation 78, 1449-58.

Czermak, B.J., Sarma, V., Bless, N.M., Schmal, H., Friedl, H.P. and Ward, P.A. (1999) In vitro and in vivo dependency of chemokine generation on C5a and TNF-alpha. J Immunol 162, 2321-5.

Danesh, J., Wheeler, J.G., Hirschfield, G.M., Eda, S., Eiriksdottir, G., Rumley, A., Lowe, G.D., Pepys, M.B. and Gudnason, V. (2004) C-reactive protein and other circulating markers of inflammation in the prediction of coronary heart disease. N Engl J Med 350, 1387-97.

de Beer, F.C., Soutar, A.K., Baltz, M.L., Trayner, I.M., Feinstein, A. and Pepys, M.B. (1982) Low density lipoprotein and very low density lipoprotein are selectively bound by aggregated C-reactive protein. J Exp Med 156, 230-42.

de Leeuw, E. and Lu, W. (2007) Human defensins: turning defense into offense? Infect Disord Drug Targets 7, 67-70.

Diepenhorst, G.M., van Gulik, T.M. and Hack, C.E. (2009) Complement-mediated ischemia-reperfusion injury: lessons learned from animal and clinical studies. Ann Surg 249, 889-99.

Endemann, D.H. and Schiffrin, E.L. (2004) Endothelial dysfunction. J Am Soc Nephrol 15, 1983-92.

Esper, R.J., Nordaby, R.A., Vilarino, J.O., Paragano, A., Cacharron, J.L. and Machado, R.A. (2006) Endothelial dysfunction: a comprehensive appraisal. Cardiovasc Diabetol 5, 4.

Flyvbjerg, A. (2010) Diabetic angiopathy, the complement system and the tumor necrosis factor superfamily. Nat Rev Endocrinol 6, 94-101.

Fosbrink, M., Niculescu, F. and Rus, H. (2005) The role of c5b-9 terminal complement complex in activation of the cell cycle and transcription. Immunol Res 31, 37-46.

Frangogiannis, N.G. (2007) Chemokines in ischemia and reperfusion. Thromb Haemost 97, 738-47.

Frangogiannis, N.G., Smith, C.W. and Entman, M.L. (2002) The inflammatory response in myocardial infarction. Cardiovasc Res 53, 31-47.

Frederiksen, P.D., Thiel, S., Larsen, C.B. and Jensenius, J.C. (2005) M-ficolin, an Innate Immune Defence Molecule, Binds Patterns of Acetyl Groups and Activates Complement. Scand J Immunol 62, 462-73.

Ganz, T. (1987) Extracellular release of antimicrobial defensins by human polymorphonuclear leukocytes. Infect Immun 55, 568-71.

Ganz, T. (2003) Defensins: antimicrobial peptides of innate immunity. Nat Rev Immunol 3, 710-20.

Gaziano, T., Reddy, K.S., Paccaud, F., Horton, S. and Chaturvedi, V. (2006) Cardiovascular Disease.

Griselli, M., Herbert, J., Hutchinson, W.L., Taylor, K.M., Sohail, M., Krausz, T. and Pepys, M.B. (1999) C-reactive protein and complement are important mediators of tissue damage in acute myocardial infarction. J Exp Med 190, 1733-40.

Groeneveld, T.W., Ramwadhdoebe, T.H., Trouw, L.A., van den Ham, D.L., van der Borden, V., Drijfhout, J.W., Hiemstra, P.S., Daha, M.R. and Roos, A. (2007) Human neutrophil peptide-1 inhibits both the classical and the lectin pathway of complement activation. Mol Immunol 44, 3608-14.

Hansen, H.H., Joensen, A.M., Riahi, S., Malczynski, J., Molenberg, D. and Ravkilde, J. (2007) Short and long-term outcome in diabetic patients with acute myocardial infarction in the invasive era. Scand Cardiovasc J 41, 19-24.

Hemingway, H., Philipson, P., Chen, R., Fitzpatrick, N.K., Damant, J., Shipley, M., Abrams, K.R., Moreno, S., McAllister, K.S., Palmer, S., Kaski, J.C., Timmis, A.D. and Hingorani, A.D. (2010) Evaluating the quality of research into a single prognostic biomarker: a systematic review and meta-analysis of 83 studies of C-reactive protein in stable coronary artery disease. PLoS Med 7, e1000286.

Higazi, A.A., Lavi, E., Bdeir, K., Ulrich, A.M., Jamieson, D.G., Rader, D.J., Usher, D.C., Kane, W., Ganz, T. and Cines, D.B. (1997) Defensin stimulates the binding of lipoprotein (a) to human vascular endothelial and smooth muscle cells. Blood 89, 4290-8.

Hill, J.H. and Ward, P.A. (1971) The phlogistic role of C3 leukotactic fragments in myocardial infarcts of rats. J Exp Med 133, 885-900.

Hirschfield, G.M. and Pepys, M.B. (2003) C-reactive protein and cardiovascular disease: new insights from an old molecule. QJM 96, 793-807.

Holmskov, U., Thiel, S. and Jensenius, J.C. (2003) Collectins and ficolins: Humoral Lectins of the Innate Immune Defense. Annu Rev Immunol 21, 547-78.

Haahr-Pedersen, S., Bjerre, M., Flyvbjerg, A., Mogelvang, R., Dominquez, H., Hansen, T.K., Galatius, S., Bech, J., Madsen, J.K., Sogaard, P. and Jensen, J.S. (2009) Level of complement activity predicts cardiac dysfunction after acute myocardial infarction treated with primary percutaneous coronary intervention. J Invasive Cardiol 21, 13-9.

Ikeda, K., Sannoh, T., Kawasaki, N., Kawasaki, T. and Yamashina, I. (1987) Serum lectin with known structure activates complement through the classical pathway. J Biol Chem 262, 7451-4.

Ito, W., Schafer, H.J., Bhakdi, S., Klask, R., Hansen, S., Schaarschmidt, S., Schofer, J., Hugo, F., Hamdoch, T. and Mathey, D. (1996) Influence of the terminal complement-complex on reperfusion injury, no-reflow and arrhythmias: a comparison between C6-competent and C6-deficient rabbits. Cardiovasc Res 32, 294-305.

Jaye, D.L. and Waites, K.B. (1997) Clinical applications of C-reactive protein in pediatrics. Pediatr Infect Dis J 16, 735-46; quiz 746-7.

Jiang, H.X., Siegel, J.N. and Gewurz, H. (1991) Binding and complement activation by C-reactive protein via the collagen-like region of C1q and inhibition of these reactions by monoclonal antibodies to C-reactive protein and C1q. J Immunol 146, 2324-30.

Johnson, E. and Hetland, G. (1991) Human umbilical vein endothelial cells synthesize functional C3, C5, C6, C8 and C9 in vitro. Scand J Immunol 33, 667-71.

Joseph, G., Tarnow, L., Astrup, A.S., Hansen, T.K., Parving, H.H., Flyvbjerg, A. and Frystyk, J. (2008) Plasma alpha-defensin is associated with cardiovascular morbidity and mortality in type 1 diabetic patients. J Clin Endocrinol Metab 93, 1470-5.

Kaplan, M.H. and Volanakis, J.E. (1974) Interaction of C-reactive protein complexes with the complement system. I. Consumption of human complement associated with the reaction of C-reactive protein with pneumococcal C-polysaccharide and with the choline phosphatides, lecithin and sphingomyelin. J Immunol 112, 2135-47.

Kaptoge, S., Di Angelantonio, E., Lowe, G., Pepys, M.B., Thompson, S.G., Collins, R. and Danesh, J. (2010) C-reactive protein concentration and risk of coronary heart disease, stroke, and mortality: an individual participant meta-analysis. Lancet 375, 132-40.

Khalil, A.A., Aziz, F.A. and Hall, J.C. (2006) Reperfusion injury. Plast Reconstr Surg 117, 1024-33.

Khot, U.N., Khot, M.B., Bajzer, C.T., Sapp, S.K., Ohman, E.M., Brener, S.J., Ellis, S.G., Lincoff, A.M. and Topol, E.J. (2003) Prevalence of conventional risk factors in patients with coronary heart disease. JAMA 290, 898-904.

Kilgore, K.S., Flory, C.M., Miller, B.F., Evans, V.M. and Warren, J.S. (1996) The membrane attack complex of complement induces interleukin-8 and monocyte chemoattractant protein-1 secretion from human umbilical vein endothelial cells. Am J Pathol 149, 953-61.

Klotman, M.E. and Chang, T.L. (2006) Defensins in innate antiviral immunity. Nat Rev Immunol 6, 447-56.

Kones, R. (2010) Rosuvastatin, inflammation, C-reactive protein, JUPITER, and primary prevention of cardiovascular disease--a perspective. Drug Des Devel Ther 4, 383-413.

Kostner, K.M., Fahti, R.B., Case, C., Hobson, P., Tate, J. and Marwick, T.H. (2006) Inflammation, complement activation and endothelial function in stable and unstable coronary artery disease. Clin Chim Acta 365, 129-34.

Kougias, P., Chai, H., Lin, P.H., Yao, Q., Lumsden, A.B. and Chen, C. (2005) Defensins and cathelicidins: neutrophil peptides with roles in inflammation, hyperlipidemia and atherosclerosis. J Cell Mol Med 9, 3-10.

Kougias, P., Chai, H., Lin, P.H., Yao, Q., Lumsden, A.B. and Chen, C. (2006) Neutrophil antimicrobial peptide alpha-defensin causes endothelial dysfunction in porcine coronary arteries. J Vasc Surg 43, 357-63.

Kyrou, I. and Tsigos, C. (2007) Stress mechanisms and metabolic complications. Horm Metab Res 39, 430-8.

Langeggen, H., Berge, K.E., Macor, P., Fischetti, F., Tedesco, F., Hetland, G., Berg, K. and Johnson, E. (2001) Detection of mRNA for the terminal complement components C5, C6, C8 and C9 in human umbilical vein endothelial cells in vitro. APMIS 109, 73-8.

Langeggen, H., Pausa, M., Johnson, E., Casarsa, C. and Tedesco, F. (2000) The endothelium is an extrahepatic site of synthesis of the seventh component of the complement system. Clin Exp Immunol 121, 69-76.

Lavie, C.J., Milani, R.V. and Ventura, H.O. (2009a) Obesity and cardiovascular disease: risk factor, paradox, and impact of weight loss. J Am Coll Cardiol 53, 1925-32.

Lavie, C.J., Milani, R.V., Verma, A. and O'Keefe, J.H. (2009b) C-reactive protein and cardiovascular diseases--is it ready for primetime? Am J Med Sci 338, 486-92.

Lennon, P.F., Collard, C.D., Morrissey, M.A. and Stahl, G.L. (1996) Complement-induced endothelial dysfunction in rabbits: mechanisms, recovery, and gender differences. Am J Physiol 270, H1924-32.

Levinson, S.S., Miller, J.J. and Elin, R.J. (2004) Poor predictive value of high-sensitivity C-reactive protein indicates need for reassessment. Clin Chem 50, 1733-5.

Madjid, M., Awan, I., Willerson, J.T. and Casscells, S.W. (2004) Leukocyte count and coronary heart disease: implications for risk assessment. J Am Coll Cardiol 44, 1945-56.

Matsushita, M., Endo, Y., Hamasaki, N. and Fujita, T. (2001) Activation of the lectin complement pathway by ficolins. Int Immunopharmacol 1, 359-63.

McManus, L.M., Kolb, W.P., Crawford, M.H., O'Rourke, R.A., Grover, F.L. and Pinckard, R.N. (1983) Complement localization in ischemic baboon myocardium. Lab Invest 48, 436-47.

Mehta, J.L. and Li, D.Y. (1999) Inflammation in ischemic heart disease: response to tissue injury or a pathogenetic villain? Cardiovasc Res 43, 291-9.

Meier-Ewert, H.K., Ridker, P.M., Rifai, N., Price, N., Dinges, D.F. and Mullington, J.M. (2001) Absence of diurnal variation of C-reactive protein concentrations in healthy human subjects. Clin Chem 47, 426-30.

Mendall, M.A., Strachan, D.P., Butland, B.K., Ballam, L., Morris, J., Sweetnam, P.M. and Elwood, P.C. (2000) C-reactive protein: relation to total mortality, cardiovascular mortality and cardiovascular risk factors in men. Eur Heart J 21, 1584-90.

Mold, C. and Morris, C.A. (2001) Complement activation by apoptotic endothelial cells following hypoxia/reoxygenation. Immunology 102, 359-64.

Muller-Eberhard, H.J. (1988) Molecular organization and function of the complement system. Annu Rev Biochem 57, 321-47.

Nassar, H., Lavi, E., Akkawi, S., Bdeir, K., Heyman, S.N., Raghunath, P.N., Tomaszewski, J. and Higazi, A.A. (2007) alpha-Defensin: link between inflammation and atherosclerosis. Atherosclerosis 194, 452-7.

Neunteufl, T., Heher, S., Katzenschlager, R., Wolfl, G., Kostner, K., Maurer, G. and Weidinger, F. (2000) Late prognostic value of flow-mediated dilation in the brachial artery of patients with chest pain. Am J Cardiol 86, 207-10.

Niculescu, F. and Rus, H. (2001) Mechanisms of signal transduction activated by sublytic assembly of terminal complement complexes on nucleated cells. Immunol Res 24, 191-9.

Oppenheim, J.J., Biragyn, A., Kwak, L.W. and Yang, D. (2003) Roles of antimicrobial peptides such as defensins in innate and adaptive immunity. Ann Rheum Dis 62 Suppl 2, ii17-21.

Pasceri, V., Cheng, J.S., Willerson, J.T. and Yeh, E.T. (2001) Modulation of C-reactive protein-mediated monocyte chemoattractant protein-1 induction in human endothelial cells by anti-atherosclerosis drugs. Circulation 103, 2531-4.

Pasceri, V., Willerson, J.T. and Yeh, E.T. (2000) Direct proinflammatory effect of C-reactive protein on human endothelial cells. Circulation 102, 2165-8.

Pearson, T.A., Mensah, G.A., Alexander, R.W., Anderson, J.L., Cannon, R.O., 3rd, Criqui, M., Fadl, Y.Y., Fortmann, S.P., Hong, Y., Myers, G.L., Rifai, N., Smith, S.C., Jr., Taubert, K., Tracy, R.P. and Vinicor, F. (2003) Markers of inflammation and cardiovascular disease: application to clinical and public health practice: A statement for healthcare professionals from the Centers for Disease Control and Prevention and the American Heart Association. Circulation 107, 499-511.

Pepys, M.B., Hirschfield, G.M., Tennent, G.A., Gallimore, J.R., Kahan, M.C., Bellotti, V., Hawkins, P.N., Myers, R.M., Smith, M.D., Polara, A., Cobb, A.J., Ley, S.V., Aquilina, J.A., Robinson, C.V., Sharif, I., Gray, G.A., Sabin, C.A., Jenvey, M.C., Kolstoe, S.E., Thompson, D. and Wood, S.P. (2006) Targeting C-reactive protein for the treatment of cardiovascular disease. Nature 440, 1217-21.

Pinckard, R.N., O'Rourke, R.A., Crawford, M.H., Grover, F.S., McManus, L.M., Ghidoni, J.J., Storrs, S.B. and Olson, M.S. (1980) Complement localization and mediation of ischemic injury in baboon myocardium. J Clin Invest 66, 1050-6.

Quinn, K., Henriques, M., Parker, T., Slutsky, A.S. and Zhang, H. (2008) Human neutrophil peptides: a novel potential mediator of inflammatory cardiovascular diseases. Am J Physiol Heart Circ Physiol 295, H1817-24.

Ridker, P.M. (2007) C-reactive protein and the prediction of cardiovascular events among those at intermediate risk: moving an inflammatory hypothesis toward consensus. J Am Coll Cardiol 49, 2129-38.

Ridker, P.M., Cannon, C.P., Morrow, D., Rifai, N., Rose, L.M., McCabe, C.H., Pfeffer, M.A. and Braunwald, E. (2005) C-reactive protein levels and outcomes after statin therapy. N Engl J Med 352, 20-8.

Ridker, P.M., Fonseca, F.A., Genest, J., Gotto, A.M., Kastelein, J.J., Khurmi, N.S., Koenig, W., Libby, P., Lorenzatti, A.J., Nordestgaard, B.G., Shepherd, J., Willerson, J.T. and Glynn, R.J. (2007) Baseline characteristics of participants in the JUPITER trial, a randomized placebo-controlled primary prevention trial of statin therapy among individuals with low low-density lipoprotein cholesterol and elevated high-sensitivity C-reactive protein. Am J Cardiol 100, 1659-64.

Ridker, P.M., Hennekens, C.H., Buring, J.E. and Rifai, N. (2000a) C-reactive protein and other markers of inflammation in the prediction of cardiovascular disease in women. N Engl J Med 342, 836-43.

Ridker, P.M., MacFadyen, J., Libby, P. and Glynn, R.J. (2010) Relation of baseline high-sensitivity C-reactive protein level to cardiovascular outcomes with rosuvastatin in the Justification for Use of statins in Prevention: an Intervention Trial Evaluating Rosuvastatin (JUPITER). Am J Cardiol 106, 204-9.

Ridker, P.M., Rifai, N., Stampfer, M.J. and Hennekens, C.H. (2000b) Plasma concentration of interleukin-6 and the risk of future myocardial infarction among apparently healthy men. Circulation 101, 1767-72.

Riedemann, N.C. and Ward, P.A. (2003) Complement in ischemia reperfusion injury. Am J Pathol 162, 363-7.

Rosamond, W., Flegal, K., Friday, G., Furie, K., Go, A., Greenlund, K., Haase, N., Ho, M., Howard, V., Kissela, B., Kittner, S., Lloyd-Jones, D., McDermott, M., Meigs, J., Moy, C., Nichol, G., O'Donnell, C.J., Roger, V., Rumsfeld, J., Sorlie, P., Steinberger, J., Thom, T., Wasserthiel-Smoller, S. and Hong, Y. (2007) Heart disease and stroke statistics--2007 update: a report from the American Heart Association Statistics Committee and Stroke Statistics Subcommittee. Circulation 115, e69-171.

Ross, R. (1999) Atherosclerosis--an inflammatory disease. N Engl J Med 340, 115-26.

Rowe, I.F., Soutar, A.K., Trayner, I.M., Thompson, G.R. and Pepys, M.B. (1984) Circulating human C-reactive protein binds very low density lipoproteins. Clin Exp Immunol 58, 237-44.

Ryden, L., Standl, E., Bartnik, M., Van den Berghe, G., Betteridge, J., de Boer, M.J., Cosentino, F., Jonsson, B., Laakso, M., Malmberg, K., Priori, S., Ostergren, J., Tuomilehto, J., Thrainsdottir, I., Vanhorebeek, I., Stramba-Badiale, M., Lindgren, P., Qiao, Q., Priori, S.G., Blanc, J.J., Budaj, A., Camm, J., Dean, V., Deckers, J., Dickstein, K., Lekakis, J., McGregor, K., Metra, M., Morais, J., Osterspey, A., Tamargo, J., Zamorano, J.L., Deckers, J.W., Bertrand, M., Charbonnel, B., Erdmann, E., Ferrannini, E., Flyvbjerg, A., Gohlke, H., Juanatey, J.R., Graham, I., Monteiro, P.F., Parhofer, K., Pyorala, K., Raz, I., Schernthaner, G., Volpe, M. and Wood, D. (2007) Guidelines on diabetes, pre-diabetes, and cardiovascular diseases: executive summary. The Task Force on Diabetes and Cardiovascular Diseases of the European Society of Cardiology (ESC) and of the European Association for the Study of Diabetes (EASD). Eur Heart J 28, 88-136.

Saraheimo, M., Forsblom, C., Pettersson-Fernholm, K., Flyvbjerg, A., Groop, P.H. and Frystyk, J. (2008) Increased levels of alpha-defensin (-1, -2 and -3) in type 1 diabetic patients with nephropathy. Nephrol Dial Transplant 23, 914-8.

Shine, B., de Beer, F.C. and Pepys, M.B. (1981) Solid phase radioimmunoassays for human C-reactive protein. Clin Chim Acta 117, 13-23.

Siegel, J., Rent, R. and Gewurz, H. (1974) Interactions of C-reactive protein with the complement system. I. Protamine-induced consumption of complement in acute phase sera. J Exp Med 140, 631-47.

St-Pierre, A.C., Cantin, B., Bergeron, J., Pirro, M., Dagenais, G.R., Despres, J.P. and Lamarche, B. (2005) Inflammatory markers and long-term risk of ischemic heart disease in men A 13-year follow-up of the Quebec Cardiovascular Study. Atherosclerosis 182, 315-21.

Stahl, G.L., Reenstra, W.R. and Frendl, G. (1995) Complement-mediated loss of endothelium-dependent relaxation of porcine coronary arteries. Role of the terminal membrane attack complex. Circ Res 76, 575-83.

Thiel, S., Vorup-Jensen, T., Stover, C.M., Schwaeble, W., Laursen, S.B., Poulsen, K., Willis, A.C., Eggleton, P., Hansen, S., Holmskov, U., Reid, K.B. and Jensenius, J.C. (1997) A second serine protease associated with mannan-binding lectin that activates complement. Nature 386, 506-10.

Urbonaviciene, G., Frystyk, J., Flyvbjerg, A., Urbonavicius, S., Henneberg, E.W. and Lindholt, J.S. (2011) Markers of inflammation in relation to long-term cardiovascular mortality in patients with lower-extremity peripheral arterial disease. Int J Cardiol.

Vakeva, A., Morgan, B.P., Tikkanen, I., Helin, K., Laurila, P. and Meri, S. (1994) Time course of complement activation and inhibitor expression after ischemic injury of rat myocardium. Am J Pathol 144, 1357-68.

Vakeva, A.P., Agah, A., Rollins, S.A., Matis, L.A., Li, L. and Stahl, G.L. (1998) Myocardial infarction and apoptosis after myocardial ischemia and reperfusion: role of the terminal complement components and inhibition by anti-C5 therapy. Circulation 97, 2259-67.

Vinten-Johansen, J. (2004) Involvement of neutrophils in the pathogenesis of lethal myocardial reperfusion injury. Cardiovasc Res 61, 481-97.

Walport, M.J. (2001) Complement. First of two parts. N Engl J Med 344, 1058-66.

Walsh, M.C., Bourcier, T., Takahashi, K., Shi, L., Busche, M.N., Rother, R.P., Solomon, S.D., Ezekowitz, R.A. and Stahl, G.L. (2005) Mannose-binding lectin is a regulator of inflammation that accompanies myocardial ischemia and reperfusion injury. J Immunol 175, 541-6.

Wang, T.J., Gona, P., Larson, M.G., Tofler, G.H., Levy, D., Newton-Cheh, C., Jacques, P.F., Rifai, N., Selhub, J., Robins, S.J., Benjamin, E.J., D'Agostino, R.B. and Vasan, R.S. (2006) Multiple biomarkers for the prediction of first major cardiovascular events and death. N Engl J Med 355, 2631-9.

Yasojima, K., Kilgore, K.S., Washington, R.A., Lucchesi, B.R. and McGeer, P.L. (1998a) Complement gene expression by rabbit heart: upregulation by ischemia and reperfusion. Circ Res 82, 1224-30.

Yasojima, K., Schwab, C., McGeer, E.G. and McGeer, P.L. (1998b) Human heart generates complement proteins that are upregulated and activated after myocardial infarction. Circ Res 83, 860-9.

Yasojima, K., Schwab, C., McGeer, E.G. and McGeer, P.L. (2001) Generation of C-reactive protein and complement components in atherosclerotic plaques. Am J Pathol 158, 1039-51.

Yudkin, J.S., Stehouwer, C.D., Emeis, J.J. and Coppack, S.W. (1999) C-reactive protein in healthy subjects: associations with obesity, insulin resistance, and endothelial dysfunction: a potential role for cytokines originating from adipose tissue? Arterioscler Thromb Vasc Biol 19, 972-8.

Zacho, J., Tybjaerg-Hansen, A., Jensen, J.S., Grande, P., Sillesen, H. and Nordestgaard, B.G. (2008) Genetically elevated C-reactive protein and ischemic vascular disease. N Engl J Med 359, 1897-908.

Zhang, M., Michael, L.H., Grosjean, S.A., Kelly, R.A., Carroll, M.C. and Entman, M.L. (2006a) The role of natural IgM in myocardial ischemia-reperfusion injury. J Mol Cell Cardiol 41, 62-7.

Zhang, M., Takahashi, K., Alicot, E.M., Vorup-Jensen, T., Kessler, B., Thiel, S., Jensenius, J.C., Ezekowitz, R.A., Moore, F.D. and Carroll, M.C. (2006b) Activation of the lectin pathway by natural IgM in a model of ischemia/reperfusion injury. J Immunol 177, 4727-34.

Zimmerman, G.A., McIntyre, T.M., Prescott, S.M. and Otsuka, K. (1990) Brief review: molecular mechanisms of neutrophil binding to endothelium involving platelet-activating factor and cytokines. J Lipid Mediat 2 Suppl, S31-43.

Zwaka, T.P., Hombach, V. and Torzewski, J. (2001) C-reactive protein-mediated low density lipoprotein uptake by macrophages: implications for atherosclerosis. Circulation 103, 1194-7.

Cardiac Biomarkers

Sadip Pant[1], Abhishek Deshmukh[1], Pritam Neupane[2],
M.P. Kavin Kumar[3] and C.S. Vijayashankar[4]
[1]University of Arkansas For Medical Sciences, Little Rock, AR
[2]Medical College of Georgia, Augusta, GA
[3]Department of Internal Medicine, Priya Hospital-Heart and
Diabetic Care Tamilnadu
[4]Apollo Hospitals Greams Road, Chennai, Tamilnadu
[1,2]USA
[3,4]India

1. Introduction

1950's: Clinical reports that transaminases released from dying myocytes could be detected via laboratory testing, aiding in the diagnosis of myocardial infarction. The race to define clinical markers to aid in the diagnosis, prognosis, and risk stratification of patients with potential cardiovascular disease begins. Initial serum markers included AST, LDH, total CK and α-hydroxybutyrate. These enzymes are all released in varying amounts by dying myocytes. Lack of sensitivity and specificity for cardiac muscle necrosis fuels continued research.

1960's:CK known to be released during muscle necrosis (including cardiac).Quantitative assays were cumbersome and difficult to perform. Total CK designed as a fast, reproducible spectrophotometric assay in the late 1960's.CK isoenzymes are subsequently described: MM, MB and BB fractions.

In 1970's MB fraction noted to be elevated in and highly specific for acute MI.

CKMB now measured via a highly sensitive monoclonal antibody assay. It was felt for a time that quantitative CKMB determination could be used to enzymatically measure the size of an infarct. This has been complicated by release of additional enzymes during reperfusion. As CK-MB assays become more sensitive, researchers come to the paradoxical realization that it too is not totally cardiac specific. The MB fraction is determined to be expressed in skeletal muscle, particularly during the process of muscle regeneration and the search for cardiac specificity continues.

Research turns towards isolation of and development of assays for sarcomeric proteins. Myosin light chains were originally isolated and then subsequently abandoned because of specificity issues. Troponin I first described as a biomarker specific for AMI in 1987; Troponin T in 1989. Now troponins are the biochemical "gold standard" for the diagnosis of acute myocardial infarction via consensus of ESC/ACC.

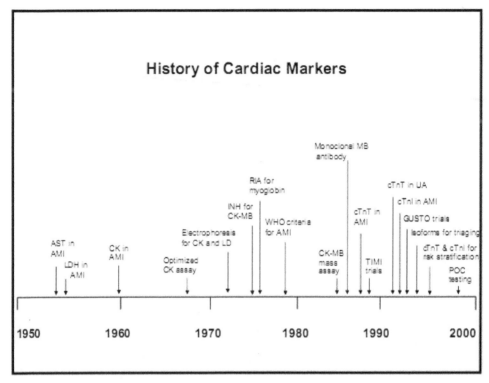

Fig. 1. Timeline showing landmark events in the development of cardiac biomarkers

1.1 Cardiac Markers: What are we looking at?

A biomarker is defined as a measurable substance or parameter that is an indicator of an underlying biological or pathological process. Therefore, depending on the underlying process that we are referring to, the cardiac markers can be classified as markers of necrosis, markers of ischemia and markers of inflammation. The features of an ideal cardiac marker would be:

- High sensitivity and specificity
- Rise and fall rapidly after ischemia
- Able to perform reliably and uniformly
- Be simple to perform
- Have turnaround time <60 min
- Not influenced by functioning of other organs, in particular, functioning of kidney.

Therefore, cardiac marker is an umbrella term which is used to define present day used necrosis markers as well as all the upstream markers of necrosis studied/under study including proinflammatory cytokines, cellular adhesion molecules, acute phase reactants, plaque destabilization biomarkers, plaque rupture biomarker and prenecrosis ischemia biomarkers. This can be simply visualized with the help of following flow diagram:

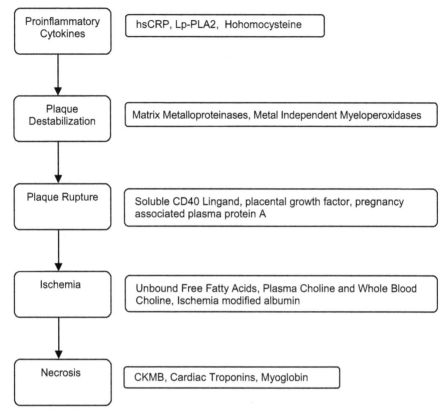

Fig. 2. Flowchart showing significance of biomarkers at various levels in the pathogenesis of acute coronary syndrome

1.2 Markers of cardiac necrosis

Cardiac markers are used in the diagnosis and risk stratification of patients with chest pain and suspected acute coronary syndrome (ACS). The cardiac troponins, in particular, have become the cardiac markers of choice for patients with ACS. Indeed, cardiac troponin is central to the definition of acute myocardial infarction (MI) in the consensus guidelines from the American College of Cardiology (ACC) and the European Society of Cardiology.

Older Definition of Myocardial Infarction- WHO 1979

1. Definite acute myocardial infarction-Definite acute myocardial infarction is diagnosed in the presence of unequivocal EKG changes and/or unequivocal enzyme changes; the history may be typical or atypical.
2. Possible acute myocardial infarction-Possible acute myocardial infarction is diagnosed when serial, equivocal ECG changes persist more than 24 hours, with or without equivocal enzyme changes; the history may be typical or atypical.
3. Old myocardial infarction-Old myocardial infarction is usually diagnosed on an unequivocal ECG in the absence of a history or enzymatic signs of acute myocardial

infarction. If there are no residual ECG changes, the diagnosis may be based on earlier, typical ECGs or on the presence of prior unequivocal serum enzyme changes.

Redefinition of Myocardial Infarction- Joint Task Force of the European Society of Cardiology, American College of Cardiology Foundation, the American Heart Association, and the World Health Federation (ESC/ACCF/AHA/WHF) 2007

A typical rise and/or gradual fall (troponin) or more rapid rise and fall (CK-MB) of biochemical markers of myocardial necrosis, with at least one of the following is required:

- Ischemic symptoms
- Development of pathologic Q waves on the ECG
- ECG changes indicative of ischemia (ST segment elevation or depression)
- Imaging evidence of new loss of viable myocardium or a new regional wall motion abnormality.

In addition, pathologic findings (generally at autopsy) of an acute MI are accepted criteria.

Markers of cardiac necrosis have come a long way since 1950s. Some of the markers used in the past are no longer in use today. Current markers and those used in the past have been outlined in the table below. Those used in the past are not discussed separately further.

Current Cardiac Markers	Cardiac Markers of the Past
• CK-MB	• Total CK Activity
• Myoglobin	• Aspartate Aminotransferase Activity
• CKMB Isoforms	• Lactate Dehydrogenase Activity
• Troponin I and T	• LD1/LD2 Ratio

Table 1. Various present day and past cardiac biomarkers

2. Creatine kinase

The enzyme creatinine kinase (formerly referred to as creatinine phosphokinase) exists as three isoenzyme forms: CK-MM, CK- MB, and CK-BB. These isoenzymes are found in the cytosol and facilitate the egress of high energy phosphates into and out of mitochondria.

CK: Dimer composed of 2 monomers: M (43,000 Da) and B (44,500 Da)---- > CK BB or CK MB or CK MM
Role: Creatine + ATP <---> ADP + Phosphocreatine + Energy (muscular contraction)
CK BB : Increased in neurological diseases ; prostatectomy; digestive cancers
CK MB : Increased with AMI
CK MM :Increased in myopathy, hypothyroidism, polymyositis, rhabdomyolysis, muscle trauma, intensive exercise, AMI

Table 2. Isoenzymes of Creatinine Kinase

Distribution of CK: Creatine Kinase (CK) isoenzyme activity is distributed in a number of tissues. The percentage of CK-MB fraction found in the heart is higher than in most other tissues. However, sensitive radioimmunoassays are able to detect small amounts of B chain protein in skeletal muscle, and some muscles have been reported to contain up to 10 percent B chain protein. Most muscles have much more CK per gram than heart tissue .As a result, despite containing only a small percent of B chain protein, skeletal muscle breakdown can lead to absolute increases in CK-MB in the plasma. Therefore, skeletal muscle damage can confound the diagnosis of an MI, as CK-MB can be released. The following are examples:

- Myocardial injury after cardiopulmonary resuscitation
- Cardioversion
- Defibrillation
- Cardiac and non-cardiac surgical procedures
- Blunt chest trauma with possible cardiac contusion
- Cocaine abuse

Total CK, CK-MB and CK-MB to Total CK ratio: Since CK is widely distributed in tissues, elevations in total serum CK lack specificity for cardiac damage, which improves with measurement of the MB fraction. The normal range of CK also varies considerably; a twofold or greater increase in the CK concentration is required for diagnosis. This criterion can be problematic in older individuals who, because of their lower muscle mass, may have low baseline serum total CK and, during MI, may have elevated serum CK-MB with values of total CK that rise but remain within the normal range. For these reasons, total CK has not been used in the diagnosis of myocardial damage for years. CK-MB has high specificity for cardiac tissue and was the preferred marker of cardiac injury for many years. An elevated CK-MB is relatively specific for myocardial injury, particularly in patients with ischemic symptoms when skeletal muscle damage is not present. Assays for CK-MB can be performed easily and rapidly. Most assays measure CK-MB mass; such measurements are more sensitive than activity assays. The relative index calculated by the ratio of CK-MB (mass) to total CK can assist in differentiating false-positive elevations of CK-MB arising from skeletal muscle. A ratio of less than 3 is consistent with a skeletal muscle source, while ratios greater than 5 are indicative of a cardiac source. Ratios between 3 and 5 represent a gray zone. No definitive diagnosis can be established without serial determinations to detect a rise. Studies to evaluate the CK-MB relative index compared with the absolute CK-MB have revealed increase in specificity but with a loss of sensitivity. The CK-MB/CK relative index is useful if patients have only an MI or only skeletal muscle injury, but not if they have both. In the combined setting of acute MI and skeletal muscle injury (rhabdomyolysis, heavy exercise, polymyositis), the fall in sensitivity is significant. It is worth noting that the diagnosis of acute MI must not be based on an elevated relative index alone, because the relative index may be elevated in clinical settings when either the total CK or the CK-MB is within normal limits. The relative index is only clinically useful when both the total CK and the CK-MB levels are increased.

Timing of Release: Creatinine Kinase starts rising in the blood 4-6 hours after the onset of chest pain. It peaks at 10-24 hours and then returns to normal after 48-72 hours. Since CK levels return to baseline 48 to 72 hours after infarction, it can be used to detect reinfarction. New elevations that occur after normalization are indicative of recurrent injury, again with the caveats in regard to sensitivity and specificity indicated above. However, for these reasons, CK-MB cannot be used for late diagnosis.

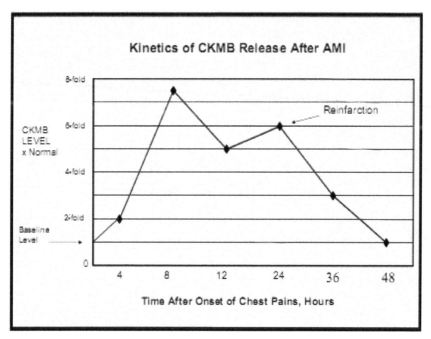

Fig. 3. Kinetics of CKMB release after AMI

Sensitivity and Specificity of CKMB: In AMI, CKMB usually is evident at 4 to 8 hours, peaks at 15 to 24 hours (mean peak=16×normal) with sensitivity and specificity >97% within the first 48 hours. By 72 hours, two thirds of patients still show some increase in CK-MB. Sampling every 6 hours is more likely to identify a peak value. False negative results may be caused by poor sample timing (e.g. only once in 24 hours or sampling <4 hours or >72 hours after AMI). Similarly, false positive may be caused by a variety of factors including but not limited to myocardial injury after cardiopulmonary resuscitation, cardioversion, defibrillation, cardiac and non-cardiac surgical procedures, blunt chest trauma with possible cardiac contusion and cocaine abuse.

CK and coronary reperfusion :The time to peak CK levels and the slope of CK-MB release can be used to assess whether reperfusion has occurred after fibrinolysis and, when used in conjunction with clinical variables, can predict whether TIMI 0 or 1 and TIMI 2 or 3 grade flow is present. The 2004 task force of the ACC/AHA concluded that serial measurements of CK-MB can be useful to provide supportive noninvasive evidence of reperfusion after fibrinolysis (class IIa recommendation). However, it should be noted that CK-MB criteria cannot identify the presence of TIMI 3 flow, which is the only level of perfusion associated with improved survival after fibrinolysis. Thus, many may elect invasive evaluation despite biomarker evidence of reperfusion. The 2004 ACC/AHA task force recommended specific guidelines for the diagnosis of reinfarction after an acute ST elevation MI. Within the first 18 hours of the initial MI, a recurrent elevation in CK-MB concentration alone should not be relied upon to diagnose reinfarction, but should be accompanied by recurrent ST segment elevation on ECG and at least one other supporting criterion (such as recurrent chest pain or hemodynamic decompensation). For patients more than 18 hours from the initial MI, a biomarker rise and at least one additional criterion is sufficient for the diagnosis. Similar criteria were established for patients presenting with possible reinfarction after percutaneous coronary intervention or coronary artery bypass grafting.

3. Cardiac Troponins

Cardiac Troponins (cTn) control the calcium-mediated interaction of actin and myosin. It exists in three isoforms: troponin C, troponin I and troponin T. Troponin C exists in all muscle tissues. cTnI is however, completely specific for the heart. cTnT released in small amounts by skeletal muscles, though clinical assays do not detect skeletal TnT. Both have cytosolic or early releasable and structural pools, with most existing in the structural pool. They are more specific compared to CKMB in detection of infarction and are the preferred biomarker for the diagnosis of acute MI (Class I recommendation from the ACC/AHA task force on diagnosis of AMI).

Characteristics	Troponin C	Troponin I	Troponin T
Weight	18 KD	26.5 KD	39 KD
Function	Calcium binding subunit	Actomyosin-ATP-inhibiting subunit	Anchors troponin complex to the tropomyosin strand
Cardiac Specificity	None	Yes	Yes

Table 3. Troponin Characteristics. KD: Kilo Dalton

3.1 Timing of release

Cardiac troponins begin rising in the blood 4-6 hours post infarction (same time as CKMB). It peaks in 12-24 hours but may take weeks to return to normal. The timing of release, peak and normal return as compared to CKMB has been presented in a graphical form below.

3.2 Sensitivity and specificity of cardiac troponins

Cardiac troponins are as sensitive as CK-MB during the first 48 hours after acute myocardial infarction. The sensitivity is 33% from 0-2 hours, 50% from 2-4 hours, 75% from 4-8 hours and approaching 100% from 8 hours after onset of chest pain. The specificity is close to 100%. Troponin elevations have been reported in a variety of clinical scenarios other than acute coronary syndromes. The following is a list of some of the causes for the elevation of troponin in the absence of a thrombotic occlusion of the coronary artery:

- Tachy- or bradyarrhythmias, or heart block
- Critically ill patients, especially with diabetes, respiratory failure or sepsis
- Hypertrophic cardiomyopathy
- Coronary vasospasm
- Acute neurological disease, including stroke or subarachnoid hemorrhage

- Cardiac contusion or other trauma including surgery, ablation, pacing, implantable cardioverter-defibrillator shocks, cardioversion, endomyocardial biopsy, cardiac surgery, following interventional closure of atrial septal defects
- Rhabdomyolysis with cardiac injury
- Congestive heart failure - acute and chronic
- Pulmonary embolism, severe pulmonary hypertension
- Renal failure
- Aortic dissection
- Aortic valve disease
- Apical ballooning syndrome - Takotsubo Cardiomyopathy
- Infiltrative diseases (ie, amyloidosis, hemochromatosis, sarcoidosis, and scleroderma)
- Inflammatory diseases (ie, myocarditis or myocardial extension of endo-/pericarditis, Kawasaki disease)
- Drug toxicity or toxins (ie, adriamycin, 5-flurouracil, herceptin, snake venom)
- Burns, especially if affecting >25 percent of body surface area
- Extreme exertion
- Transplant vasculopathy

The 2007 joint ESC/ACCF/AHA/WHF task force recommends that an elevated value of cardiac troponin, in the absence of clinical evidence of ischemia, should prompt a search for other causes of myocardial necrosis as listed above.

3.3 Troponin assays

The skeletal and cardiac isoforms of troponin T and troponin I are distinct, and skeletal isoforms are not detected by the monoclonal antibody-based assays currently in use. This specificity for cardiac isoforms is the basis for the clinical utility of cTnT and cTnI assays. Contemporary troponin assays are quite sensitive and can detect very small amounts of myocardial necrosis (<1 g). Troponin C is not used clinically because both cardiac and smooth muscle share troponin C isoforms. The ESC/ACC recommended that the diagnosis of MI be based on troponin levels in excess of the 99th percentile of a reference control group. As cTnT and cTnI levels are undetectable in most normal subjects, the 99th percentile is very low (eg, 0.04 to 0.5 micrograms/L). However, most assays are imprecise at this low level, and so it has been recommended that the definition of MI be raised to that value at which a specific assay has a coefficient of variation of 10 percent or less. New guidelines embrace 99th percentile for two reasons. This level is also low (0.1 to 1.2 micrograms/L), but higher than the 99th percentile standard. Due to variations in assay precision and individual laboratory policies, the upper limit of normal varies between laboratories, but in all cases is above the 99th percentile.

3.4 Point-of-care assays

The National Academy of Clinical Biochemistry (NACB) recommendations specify that cardiac markers be available on an immediate basis 24 h/d, 7 d/wk, with a turnaround time of 1 hour. Point-of-care (POC) devices that provide rapid results should be considered in hospitals whose laboratories cannot meet these guidelines. POC assays for CK-MB, myoglobin, and the cardiac troponins TnI and TnT are available. Only qualitative TnT assays are available as POC tests, but both quantitative and qualitative POC TnI assays are currently marketed. In a multicenter trial, the time to positivity was significantly faster for the POC device than for the local laboratory (2.5 h vs 3.4 h).In another multicenter study, which evaluated the i-STAT POC TnI assay in comparison with the central laboratory in 2000 patients with suspected ACS, POC testing reduced the length of stay by approximately 25 minutes for patients who were discharged from the ED. The sensitivity of current POC assays coupled with the benefit of rapid turnaround time make the POC assays attractive clinical tools in the ED.

3.5 Prognostic value of cardiac troponins

In addition to its use in the diagnosis of MI, an elevated troponin level can identify patients at high risk for adverse cardiac events. Specifically, data from a meta-analysis indicated that an elevated troponin level in patients without ST-segment elevation is associated with a nearly 4-fold increase in the cardiac mortality rate. In patients without ST-segment elevation who were being considered for thrombolytic therapy, initial TnI levels on admission correlated with mortality at 6 weeks, but CK-MB levels were not predictive of adverse cardiac events and had no prognostic value. Other studies revealed that an elevated troponin level at baseline was an independent predictor of mortality, even in patients with chest pain and acute MI with ST-segment elevation who were eligible for reperfusion therapy. Finally, the TIMI IIIB, GUSTO IIa, GUSTO IV ACS, and FRISC trial all demonstrated a direct correlation between the level of TnI or TnT and the mortality rate and adverse cardiac event rate in ACS.

3.6 High Sensitive Troponin (hsTroponin)

High-sensitive assay is one which has a total imprecision of less than 10% at the 99th percentile and some would propose also being able to quantitate over 50% of normal values below that 99th percentile. High-sensitive cTn assays have two differentiating features from contemporary cTn assays: 1) detection of cTn in healthy persons and 2) a precise definition of what is "normal" (= the 99th percentile). Recent multicenter studies have shown that high-sensitive cTn assays improve the early diagnosis of acute myocardial infarction (AMI). To achieve the best clinical use, cTn has to be interpreted as a quantitative variable. Rising and/or falling levels differentiate acute from chronic cardiomyocyte necrosis. The term "troponin-positive" should therefore be avoided. "Detectable" levels will become the norm and have to be clearly differentiated from "elevated" levels. The differential diagnosis of a small amount of cardiomyocyte necrosis and therefore mild elevation of cTn is broad and includes acute and chronic cardiac disorders. The differential diagnosis of a large amount of cardiomyocyte necrosis and therefore substantial elevation of cTn is much smaller and largely restricted to AMI, myocarditis and Takotsubo cardiomyopathy. Two large prospective multicenter studies showed that sensitive and high-sensitive cTn assays have a higher diagnostic accuracy compared to contemporary cTn assays at presentation, in the diagnosis of AMI. Earlier "rule in" may reduce morbidity by allowing earlier revascularization, earlier transfer to the coronary care unit, and earlier initiation of evidence-based AMI treatment. Nonetheless, the improvement in sensitivity is at the expense of specificity. There is still considerable controversy in regard to how to use these assays to detect acute events such as AMI. Hence, at this time it has not been approved for clinical use and is yet in research phase.

4. Myoglobin

Myoglobin is a heme protein found in skeletal and cardiac muscle that has attracted considerable interest as an early marker of MI. Its low molecular weight accounts for its early release profile: myoglobin typically rises 2-4 hours after onset of infarction, peaks at 6-12 hours, and returns to normal within 24-36 hours. Rapid myoglobin assays are available, but overall, they have a lack of cardiospecificity. Serial sampling every 1-2 hours can increase the sensitivity and specificity; a rise of 25-40% over 1-2 hours is strongly suggestive of acute MI. However, in most studies, myoglobin only achieved 90% sensitivity for acute MI, so the negative predictive value of myoglobin is not high enough to exclude the diagnosis of acute MI. The original studies that evaluated myoglobin used the WHO definition of acute MI that was based on a CK-MB standard. With the adoption of a troponin standard for acute MI in the ACC/ESC definition, the sensitivity of myoglobin for acute MI is substantially reduced. This significantly diminishes its utility, and a number of studies have indicated that contemporary cardiac troponin assays render the use of myoglobin measurements unnecessary.

Conditions where myoglobin increases	Conditions where myoglobin does not increase
Acute myocardial infarction	Non cardiac chest pain
Vigorous exercise	Mild to moderate exercise
Open heart surgery	CHF without acute myocardial infarction
Rhabdomyolysis	Cardiac catheterization
Progressive muscular dystrophy	
Shock	
Renal Failure	

Table 4. Serum myoglobin in various clinical conditions

4.1 Timing of release, peak and return to baseline of various cardiac markers

CAD is highly prevalent in patients with CKD, making interpretation of cardiac markers important. Despite this, interpretation of elevated cardiac enzymes in patients with renal failure is often confusing at best. Elevations in serum troponin often observed in asymptomatic patients with chronic kidney disease. Even using the most conservative cutoff values, a disproportionate number of patients still have elevated troponins. The mechanism for this is unclear. In a 2002 study in *Circulation*, 733 asymptomatic patients with ESRD were evaluated. Using conservative cutoff values,

-    82% had elevated cTnT
-    6% had elevated cTnI

Of those 733 asymptomatic patients on HD, 2-year mortality rates were 52% in those with cTnI ≥0.1 µg/dL .These data have been corroborated in a number of smaller studies in similar populations. Serial measurements are helpful in the setting of possible ACS. cTnI appears to be much less likely to be associated with false positives in the CKD population than cTnT, making it the preferred biomarker in this setting.

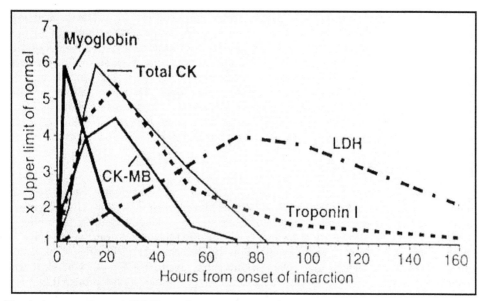

Fig. 4. A comparison of CKMB, cardiac troponins and myoglobin.

4.2 Markers of inflammation

Acute coronary syndromes are caused by vulnerable plaques. It is thought that one of the driving forces causing atheromatous plaques to rupture or erode, causing a cascade of events leading to coronary artery occlusion, is inflammation in the plaques. In this section cardiac inflammatory markers are dealt with which is at the verge of entering into clinical practice as tool for diagnosing and predicting future cardiovascular events at earlier stage and for risk stratification. Highly Sensitive Creative Protein (hsCRP), Myeloperoxidase (MPO), Matrix Metalloproteinases (MMP), Pregnancy Associated Protein A(PAPP-A),Placenta Growth Factor(PlGF) are reviewed.

4.3 C-Reactive protein (CRP)

C Reactive Protein is an acute phase reactant synthesized in liver and is elevated in inflammatory conditions. Once ligand-bound, CRP can activate the classical compliment pathway, stimulate phagocytosis and bind to immunoglobulin receptors. "High-sensitivity" only means that the concentration of CRP was determined using an assay designed to measure very low levels of CRP. The American Heart Association has defined risk groups as follows: Low risk: less than 1.0 mg/L, Average risk: 1.0 to 3.0 mg/L and High risk: above 3.0 mg/L. Two assays averaged fasting or non fasting, and optimally 2 weeks apart, provide a more stable estimate of level of this marker. If a level is greater than 10 mg/L is identified, there should be a search initiated for an obvious source of infection or inflammation, which could obscure any prediction of coronary risk that might be attributed to the elevated level. The landmark study by Liuzzo et al. showed that patients presenting with unstable angina and elevated plasma concentrations of CRP had a higher rate of death, MI and need for re-vascularisation compared with patients without elevated concentrations. In more recent trials, other investigators have confirmed the increased risk in ACS associated with higher CRP concentrations. In each of the above studies, the predictive value of CRP was independent of, and additive to, cardiac troponin. More importantly, CRP was found to have prognostic value even among patients with negative cardiac troponin and no evidence of myocyte necrosis. Methodological issues have however been highlighted and the independence between CRP and troponin release questioned. Therefore , although many studies have suggested that low-grade hsCRP elevations are independently associated with coronary risk, more complete evidence is needed to validate the use of hs-CRP as a risk assessment tool in general practice and as a target for therapy in individual patients .

4.4 Myeloperoxidase (MPO)

Myeloperoxidase (MPO) is a hemoprotein that is abundantly expressed in polymorphonuclear cells (neutrophils) and secreted during their activation. The presence of a peroxidase in the cytoplasmic granules of leukocytes was suggested at the beginning of 20th century but it was the early 1940s that it was purified for the first time. MPO plays an important role in neutrophil microbicidal action through catalyzing chloride ion oxidation to hypochlorous acid, which is a potent antimicrobial agent. On the other hand, it was demonstrated that MPO causes oxidative modification of low density lipoprotein (LDL) to a high uptake form that is considered to be a key event in the promotion of atherogenesis. Hence myeloperoxidase is believed to participate in the initiation and progression of cardiovascular diseases. MPO possesses potent proinflammatory properties and may contribute directly to tissue injury.

In a study consisted of patients diagnosed with ACS and other heart disease or unspecified chest pain, considerably higher MPO concentrations were demonstrated in the troponin-negative ACS patients on admission who became troponin-positive after 6h. This suggests that level of MPO possessed remarkably higher sensitivity than assessment of cTnI alone in all patients with ACS. MPO levels are associated with the presence of angiographically proven coronary atherosclerosis. In addition to clinical history and other tools MPO has been approved by FDA as cardiac biomarker to evaluate the patients with chest pain and at high risk for coronary artery disease.

4.5 Matrix metalloproteinases (MMP)

MMP are endogenous zinc dependent endopeptidases required for structural integrity of extracellular matrix of myocardium. TIMP (Tissue Inhibitors of Metalloproteinases) regulates MMP. MMPs may degrade myocardial ECM leading to the development of LV dilatation and heart failure and their inhibition in experimental models of AMI has been associated with reduced LV dilatation and wall stress. In a study of patients with acute myocardial infarction, TIMP-1 and MMP-9 correlated with echocardiographic parameters of LV dysfunction and remodelling after AMI and identified patients at risk of subsequent LV remodeling and associated with severe extensive CAD.

4.6 Placental Growth Factors (PGF)

Placental Growth Factor is a member of VEGF (vascular endothelial growth factor) subfamily - a key molecule in angiogenesis and vasculogenesis, in particular during the embryogenesis. Placental growth factor expression within human atherosclerotic lesions is associated with plaque inflammation and neovascular growth. Recent studies established the role of different inflammatory markers such as hsCRP, sr amyloid A, IL-6 not only gets elevated during acute coronary syndrome (ACS) but predicts its adverse outcomes. PGF was recently shown that it is upregulated in all forms of atherosclerotic lesions. PGIF induces the following

- Vascular smooth muscle cell growth.
- Recruits macrophages into atherosclerotic lesions.
- Upregulates production of TNF alpha.
- Monocyte chemotactic protein 1 by macrophages.
- Pathological angiogenesis.

Plasma PIGF levels may be an independent inflammatory biomarker of poor outcome in patients with suspected ACS. A single initial measurement of plasma PIGF appears to extend the predictive and prognostic information gained from traditional inflammatory markers.

5. Pregnancy associated plasma protein alpha (PAPP-A)

PAPP-A was originally identified in the serum of pregnant women. PAPP-A is produced by placental tissue. Circulating PAPP-A levels increase during pregnancy and they are used in the fetal diagnosis of Down syndrome. Only recently has PAPP-A been identified in nonplacental tissues. The concentrations in the sera of nonpregnant human beings being several orders of magnitude lower than during pregnancy. The physiological role of PAPP-A is only beginning to be unraveled. PAPP-A is a high-molecular-weight, zinc-binding metalloproteinase, which acts as a specific protease of IGF binding protein-4 (IGFBP-4). There is histological evidence, using specific monoclonal antibodies, that PAPP-A is abundantly expressed in both eroded and ruptured coronary plaques, but not in stable plaques, in patients who have died suddenly of cardiac causes. Furthermore, accumulating evidence suggests that PAPP-A may play a pivotal role in the development of atherosclerosis and subsequent plaque instability in ACS patients. PAPP-A is markedly elevated in the earliest hours after the onset of symptoms in patients with STEMIs treated with heparin and primary percutaneous coronary intervention, and in animal studies, heparin administration is associated with a significant increase in PAPP-A levels, presumably because of the detachment of PAPP-A from the vessel wall. If future studies confirm that concomitant heparin administration also increases PAPP-A levels in humans, the prognostic role of PAPP-A in patients with ST elevation myocardial infarction needs to be reevaluated.

5.1 Markers of ischemia

An ideal marker is one in which there is a specific easily measurable increase that clearly aligns with a predictable outcome be it evidence of ischemia, inflammation, myocardial necrosis, plaque rupture, plaque destabilization, or heart failure. Because of the underlying shared etiologies related to the process of arteriosclerosis and the complexity of the pathological processes giving rise to adverse thrombotic outcomes, a single marker that relates to each stage is unlikely. Rather more probable would be use of multiple markers with varying decision levels to either rule-in or rule-out a clinical decision. As the understanding of the niceties between ACS, inflammation, and coronary artery process develops, the ongoing search for better cardiac markers will continue.

5.2 Ischemia modified albumin (IMA)

The only ischemia marker that has been approved by the FDA is the modified albumin (IMA) using the albumin cobalt binding test (ACB) for assessment of myocardial ischemia. IMA occurs in 2 forms: 1.in which human serum albumin (HAS) binds mostly copper and 2.in which the damage to the N-terminus prevents metal binding. Patients without ischemia have more available metal binding sites on their HSA, than those from ischemic patients. This alteration is most likely due to damage caused by oxidative free radicals prevalent during ischemic events, and resulting in altered binding of trace metals resulting in IMA. As mentioned earlier, the FDA approved method for IMA (ACB Test by Ischemia Technologies) uses cobalt in its assay. Normal HSA will bind cobalt when it is added to a sample, leaving little residual cobalt. However, IMA cannot do the same due to its altered binding site. Patients having transient ischemic episodes without parallel myocyte death increases IMA which causes less cobalt binding and more residual unbound cobalt available. This can complex with chromogen (dithiothreitol) which can be measured photometrically. It is estimated that approximately 1% to 2% of the total albumin concentration in the normal population is IMA compared to 6% to 8% in patients experiencing ischemia. The clinical utility of IMA appears to be in its negative predictive value for ischemia and ACS, particularly when used in conjunction with other tests. While the optimum cutoff for IMA for ruling out ACS is 85kU/L, the manufacturer has suggested a higher value of 100 kU/L for risk stratification. Some of the limitations to be taken into consideration includes: a. there is an overlap between the normal population and that of individuals with cardiac ischemia; b. IMA is not specific for cardiac ischemia; c. false positive can occur in patients with cirrhosis, bacterial and viral infections, advanced cancers, stroke and end-stage renal disease and d. interpretation of IMA in certain populations, including those with peripheral vascular disease and in marathon runners is not yet clear. Hence IMA appears at this time as a potential marker in certain clinical situations but a number of possible interferences may limit its utility in patients with suspected ACS.

5.3 Unbound free fatty acids

Fatty acids are essential building blocks for many lipid molecules and are energy stores that can be utilized during times of fasting or increased metabolic demand. Fatty acids exist in body as esterified form (bound to glycerol or other alcohol), non-esterified form bound to albumin, and to a much smaller extent, as an unbound soluble form. Evidence exists that unbound free fatty acids increase significantly in ischemic-related events. It is not certain as of today what role the unbound free fatty acid plays in cardiac disease. It possibly partakes in the developing necrotic process and is released as a result of cell rupture or other precipitating conditions. Currently, a fluorescent probe assay is available but its clinical utility at this time is not established.

5.4 Fatty acid binding proteins (FABPs)

Fatty acid binding proteins (FABPs) are transport proteins that carry fatty acids and other lipophilic molecules like eicosanoids and retinoids across the membranes. They occur in nine different isoforms in a predictable tissue distribution and fairly long half-life of several days. The heart-type FABP (H-FABP) is released following myocardial death within 6 hours and is not specific to the heart, similar to myoglobin. It is released to a smaller extent in skeletal muscle, distal tubular cells of the kidney, specific parts of the brain, lactating mammary glands, and the placenta. It has been found that H-FABP may perform better and reach its upper reference limit sooner than either myoglobin or troponin. A number of enzyme immunoassays are available for H-FABP testing. Its relation to ischemia and prognosis for adverse events is likely to expound in near future.

5.5 Phospholipase

Phospholipase are the enzymes that release fatty acids from the second carbon group of glycerol. They are grouped into 4 major categories: A to D. Phospholipase A2 and D have drawn much attention in their role in assessing ischemia associated coronary artery disease. Lipoprotein-associated phospholipase A_2 (Lp-PLA$_2$) also known as platelet-activating factor acetylhydrolase (PAF-AH) is a phospholipase A2 enzyme that in humans is encoded by the PLA2G7 gene. In human atherosclerotic lesions, 2 main sources of Lp-PLA$_2$ can be identified, including that which is brought into the intima bound to LDL (from the circulation), and that which is synthesized de novo by plaque inflammatory cells (macrophages, T cells, mast cells). I A meta-analysis involving a total of 79,036 participants in 32 prospective studies found that Lp-PLA$_2$ levels are positively correlated with increased risk of developing coronary heart disease and stroke. Recently, there has been a renewed interest in this molecule, not for use in cardiac assessment as it was originally approved by the FDA, but rather in stroke prediction after it was found that elevated levels of Lp-PLA2 were associated with an almost 2-fold increase in stroke in the selected population coupled with a 6-fold increase in hypertensive individuals.

Phospholipase D (PLD) is an enzyme that catalyzes the hydrolysis of membrane bound phospholipids into phosphatidic acid and choline. In addition, it is also involved in endorsement of fibrinogen binding to platelets. Increased levels of plasma (PLCHO) and whole blood choline (WBCHO) levels have been seen in tissue ischemia in patients with negative troponin values. Choline is not a marker for myocardial necrosis but indicated high-risk unstable angina in patients without acute myocardial infarction (sensitivity 86.4%, specificity 86.2%). Therefore obtaining levels of both plasma PLCHO and WBCHO may prove to be a useful aid in patients suspected of ACS.

6. Conclusion

Cardiac markers have been implicated in the diagnosis and risk stratification of patients with chest pain and suspected acute coronary syndrome (ACS). Among the markers of cardiac necrosis, troponins have become the cardiac markers of choice for patients with ACS. In fact, cardiac troponin has become central to the definition of acute myocardial infarction (MI) in the consensus guidelines from the American College of Cardiology (ACC) and the European Society of Cardiology (ESC). Current focus is on finding appropriate upstream markers which may aid in detection of myocardial ischemia and a variety of events involved in the process of pathophysiology of acute coronary syndrome especially in relation to plaque destabilization and rupture. The ideal biomarkers that offer early detection, risk stratification, selection of therapy, monitoring disease progression, and treatment efficacy remain to be elucidated.

7. References

[1] Jaffe AS, Ravkilde J, Roberts R, et al. It's time for a change to a troponin standard. Circulation 2000; 102:1216.

[2] Shave R, George KP, Atkinson G, et al. Exercise-induced cardiac troponin T release: a meta-analysis. Med Sci Sports Exerc 2007; 39:2099.

[3] Gupta S, de Lemos JA. Use and misuse of cardiac troponins in clinical practice. Prog Cardiovasc Dis 2007; 50:151.

[4] Müller-Bardorff M, Weidtmann B, Giannitsis E, et al. Release kinetics of cardiac troponin T in survivors of confirmed severe pulmonary embolism. Clin Chem 2002; 48:673.

[5] Carlson RJ, Navone A, McConnell JP, et al. Effect of myocardial ischemia on cardiac troponin I and T. Am J Cardiol 2002; 89:224.

[6] Sabatine MS, Morrow DA, de Lemos JA, et al. Detection of acute changes in circulating troponin in the setting of transient stress test-induced myocardial ischaemia using an ultrasensitive assay: results from TIMI 35. Eur Heart J 2009; 30:162.

[7] Kurz K, Giannitsis E, Zehelein J, Katus HA. Highly sensitive cardiac troponin T values remain constant after brief exercise- or pharmacologic-induced reversible myocardial ischemia. Clin Chem 2008; 54:1234.

[8] Adams JE 3rd, Abendschein DR, Jaffe AS. Biochemical markers of myocardial injury. Is MB creatine kinase the choice for the 1990s? Circulation 1993; 88:750.

[9] Katus HA, Remppis A, Scheffold T, et al. Intracellular compartmentation of cardiac troponin T and its release kinetics in patients with reperfused and nonreperfused myocardial infarction. Am J Cardiol 1991; 67:1360.

[10] Adams JE 3rd, Schechtman KB, Landt Y, et al. Comparable detection of acute myocardial infarction by creatine kinase MB isoenzyme and cardiac troponin I. Clin Chem 1994; 40:1291.

[11] Adams JE III, Bodor, GS, Davila-Roman, VG, et al. Cardiac troponin I. A marker with high specificity for cardiac injury. Circulation 1993; 88:101.

[12] Bodor GS, Porterfield D, Voss EM, et al. Cardiac troponin-I is not expressed in fetal and healthy or diseased adult human skeletal muscle tissue. Clin Chem 1995; 41:1710.

[13] Ricchiuti V, Voss EM, Ney A, et al. Cardiac troponin T isoforms expressed in renal diseased skeletal muscle will not cause false-positive results by the second generation cardiac troponin T assay by Boehringer Mannheim. Clin Chem 1998; 44:1919.

[14] Panteghini M, Pagani F, Yeo KT, et al. Evaluation of imprecision for cardiac troponin assays at low-range concentrations. Clin Chem 2004; 50:327.

[15] Apple FS, Quist HE, Doyle PJ, et al. Plasma 99th percentile reference limits for cardiac troponin and creatine kinase MB mass for use with European Society of Cardiology/American College of Cardiology consensus recommendations. Clin Chem 2003; 49:1331.

[16] Shi Q, Ling M, Zhang X, et al. Degradation of cardiac troponin I in serum complicates comparisons of cardiac troponin I assays. Clin Chem 1999; 45:1018.

[17] Labugger R, Organ L, Collier C, et al. Extensive troponin I and T modification detected in serum from patients with acute myocardial infarction. Circulation 2000; 102:1221.

[18] Heeschen C, Goldmann BU, Langenbrink L, et al. Evaluation of a rapid whole blood ELISA for quantification of troponin I in patients with acute chest pain. Clin Chem 1999; 45:1789.

[19] Katrukha AG, Bereznikova AV, Esakova TV, et al. Troponin I is released in bloodstream of patients with acute myocardial infarction not in free form but as complex. Clin Chem 1997; 43:1379.

[20] Wu AH, Feng YJ, Moore R, et al. Characterization of cardiac troponin subunit release into serum after acute myocardial infarction and comparison of assays for troponin T and I. American Association for Clinical Chemistry Subcommittee on cTnI Standardization. Clin Chem 1998; 44:1198.

[21] Thygesen K, Alpert JS, White HD, Joint ESC/ACCF/AHA/WHF Task Force for the Redefinition of Myocardial Infarction. Universal definition of myocardial infarction. Eur Heart J 2007; 28:2525.

[22] Panteghini M, Gerhardt W, Apple FS, et al. Quality specifications for cardiac troponin assays. Clin Chem Lab Med 2001; 39:175.

[23] Lee TH, Thomas EJ, Ludwig LE, et al. Troponin T as a marker for myocardial ischemia in patients undergoing major noncardiac surgery. Am J Cardiol 1996; 77:1031.

[24] Baum H, Braun S, Gerhardt W, et al. Multicenter evaluation of a second-generation assay for cardiac troponin T. Clin Chem 1997; 43:1877.

[25] Apple FS, Parvin CA, Buechler KF, et al. Validation of the 99th percentile cutoff independent of assay imprecision (CV) for cardiac troponin monitoring for ruling out myocardial infarction. Clin Chem 2005; 51:2198.

[26] Wu AH, Jaffe AS. The clinical need for high-sensitivity cardiac troponin assays for acute coronary syndromes and the role for serial testing. Am Heart J 2008; 155:208.

[27] Zethelius B, Johnston N, Venge P. Troponin I as a predictor of coronary heart disease and mortality in 70-year-old men: a community-based cohort study. Circulation 2006; 113:1071.

[28] Kavsak PA, Newman AM, Lustig V, et al. Long-term health outcomes associated with detectable troponin I concentrations. Clin Chem 2007; 53:220.

[29] Waxman DA, Hecht S, Schappert J, Husk G. A model for troponin I as a quantitative predictor of in-hospital mortality. J Am Coll Cardiol 2006; 48:1755.

[30] Schulz O, Kirpal K, Stein J, et al. Importance of low concentrations of cardiac troponins. Clin Chem 2006; 52:1614.

[31] Wu AH, Fukushima N, Puskas R, et al. Development and preliminary clinical validation of a high sensitivity assay for cardiac troponin using a capillary flow (single molecule) fluorescence detector. Clin Chem 2006; 52:2157.

[32] Kavsak PA, MacRae AR, Yerna MJ, Jaffe AS. Analytic and clinical utility of a next-generation, highly sensitive cardiac troponin I assay for early detection of myocardial injury. Clin Chem 2009; 55:573.

[33] Wilson SR, Sabatine MS, Braunwald E, et al. Detection of myocardial injury in patients with unstable angina using a novel nanoparticle cardiac troponin I assay: observations from the PROTECT-TIMI 30 Trial. Am Heart J 2009; 158:386.

[34] Venge P, Johnston N, Lindahl B, James S. Normal plasma levels of cardiac troponin I measured by the high-sensitivity cardiac troponin I access prototype assay and the impact on the diagnosis of myocardial ischemia. J Am Coll Cardiol 2009; 54:1165.

[35] Giannitsis E, Kurz K, Hallermayer K, et al. Analytical validation of a high-sensitivity cardiac troponin T assay. Clin Chem 2010; 56:254.

[36] Latini R, Masson S, Anand IS, et al. Prognostic value of very low plasma concentrations of troponin T in patients with stable chronic heart failure. Circulation 2007; 116:1242.

[37] Januzzi JL Jr, Bamberg F, Lee H, et al. High-sensitivity troponin T concentrations in acute chest pain patients evaluated with cardiac computed tomography. Circulation 2010; 121:1227.

[38] Diamond GA, Kaul S. How would the Reverend Bayes interpret high-sensitivity troponin? Circulation 2010; 121:1172.

[39] Kavsak PA, Wang X, Ko DT, et al. Short- and long-term risk stratification using a next-generation, high-sensitivity research cardiac troponin I (hs-cTnI) assay in an emergency department chest pain population. Clin Chem 2009; 55:1809.

[40] Derdeyn CP. Moyamoya disease and moyamoya syndrome. N Engl J Med 2009; 361:97; author reply 98.

[41] de Lemos JA, Drazner MH, Omland T, et al. Association of troponin T detected with a highly sensitive assay and cardiac structure and mortality risk in the general population. JAMA 2010; 304:2503.

[42] deFilippi CR, de Lemos JA, Christenson RH, et al. Association of serial measures of cardiac troponin T using a sensitive assay with incident heart failure and cardiovascular mortality in older adults. JAMA 2010; 304:2494.

[43] Katus HA, Giannitsis E, Jaffe AS, Thygesen K. Higher sensitivity troponin assays: Quo vadis? Eur Heart J 2009; 30:127.

[44] Wallace TW, Abdullah SM, Drazner MH, et al. Prevalence and determinants of troponin T elevation in the general population. Circulation 2006; 113:1958.

[45] Daniels LB, Laughlin GA, Clopton P, et al. Minimally elevated cardiac troponin T and elevated N-terminal pro-B-type natriuretic peptide predict mortality in older adults: results from the Rancho Bernardo Study. J Am Coll Cardiol 2008; 52:450.

[46] Jaffe AS. Chasing troponin: how low can you go if you can see the rise? J Am Coll Cardiol 2006; 48:1763.

[47] Mills NL, Churchhouse AM, Lee KK, et al. Implementation of a sensitive troponin I assay and risk of recurrent myocardial infarction and death in patients with suspected acute coronary syndrome. JAMA 2011; 305:1210.

[48] Saenger AK, Jaffe AS. Requiem for a heavyweight: the demise of creatine kinase-MB. Circulation 2008; 118:2200.

[49] Antman, EM, Anbe, DT, Armstrong, PW, et al. ACC/AHA guidelines for the management of patients with ST-elevation myocardial infarction. www.acc.org/qualityandscience/clinical/statements.htm (Accessed on August 24, 2006).

[50] Macrae AR, Kavsak PA, Lustig V, et al. Assessing the requirement for the 6-hour interval between specimens in the American Heart Association Classification of Myocardial Infarction in Epidemiology and Clinical Research Studies. Clin Chem 2006; 52:812.

[51] Eggers KM, Oldgren J, Nordenskjöld A, Lindahl B. Diagnostic value of serial measurement of cardiac markers in patients with chest pain: limited value of adding myoglobin to troponin I for exclusion of myocardial infarction. Am Heart J 2004; 148:574.

[52] Hollander JE, Levitt MA, Young GP, et al. Effect of recent cocaine use on the specificity of cardiac markers for diagnosis of acute myocardial infarction. Am Heart J 1998; 135:245.

[53] Reichlin T, Hochholzer W, Bassetti S, et al. Early diagnosis of myocardial infarction with sensitive cardiac troponin assays. N Engl J Med 2009; 361:858.

[54] Keller T, Zeller T, Peetz D, et al. Sensitive troponin I assay in early diagnosis of acute myocardial infarction. N Engl J Med 2009; 361:868.

[55] Jaffe, AS and Apple FS. High-sensitivity cardiac troponin: Hype, help, and reality. Clinical chemistry 2009; Dec 30. [E pub ahead of print].

[56] Antman, EM, Hand, M, Armstrong, PW, et al. 2007 focused update of the ACC/AHA 2004 Guidelines for the Management of Patients With ST-Elevation Myocardial Infarction: a report of the American College of Cardiology/American Heart Association Task Force on Practice Guidelines (Writing Group to Review New Evidence and Update the ACC/AHA 2004 Guidelines for the Management of Patients With ST-Elevation Myocardial Infarction). J Am Coll Cardiol 2008; 51:XXX. Available at: www.acc.org/qualityandscience/clinical/statements.htm (accessed September 18, 2007).

[57] deFilippi CR, Tocchi M, Parmar RJ, et al. Cardiac troponin T in chest pain unit patients without ischemic electrocardiographic changes: angiographic correlates and long-term clinical outcomes. J Am Coll Cardiol 2000; 35:1827.

[58] Ohman EM, Christenson RH, Califf RM, et al. Noninvasive detection of reperfusion after thrombolysis based on serum creatine kinase MB changes and clinical variables. TAMI 7 Study Group. Thrombolysis and Angioplasty in Myocardial Infarction. Am Heart J 1993; 126:819.

[59] Christenson RH, Ohman EM, Topol EJ, et al. Assessment of coronary reperfusion after thrombolysis with a model combining myoglobin, creatine kinase-MB, and clinical

variables. TAMI-7 Study Group. Thrombolysis and Angioplasty in Myocardial Infarction-7. Circulation 1997; 96:1776.

[60] Apple FS, Murakami MM. Cardiac troponin and creatine kinase MB monitoring during in-hospital myocardial reinfarction. Clin Chem 2005; 51:460.

[61] Babuin L, Vasile VC, Rio Perez JA, et al. Elevated cardiac troponin is an independent risk factor for short- and long-term mortality in medical intensive care unit patients. Crit Care Med 2008; 36:759.

[62] Allan JJ, Feld RD, Russell AA, et al. Cardiac troponin I levels are normal or minimally elevated after transthoracic cardioversion. J Am Coll Cardiol 1997; 30:1052.

[63] Licka M, Zimmermann R, Zehelein J, et al. Troponin T concentrations 72 hours after myocardial infarction as a serological estimate of infarct size. Heart 2002; 87:520.

[64] Panteghini M, Cuccia C, Bonetti G, et al. Single-point cardiac troponin T at coronary care unit discharge after myocardial infarction correlates with infarct size and ejection fraction. Clin Chem 2002; 48:1432.

[65] Steen H, Giannitsis E, Futterer S, et al. Cardiac troponin T at 96 hours after acute myocardial infarction correlates with infarct size and cardiac function. J Am Coll Cardiol 2006; 48:2192.

[66] Giannitsis E, Steen H, Kurz K, et al. Cardiac magnetic resonance imaging study for quantification of infarct size comparing directly serial versus single time-point measurements of cardiac troponin T. J Am Coll Cardiol 2008; 51:307.

[67] Vasile VC, Babuin L, Giannitsis E, et al. Relationship of MRI-determined infarct size and cTnI measurements in patients with ST-elevation myocardial infarction. Clin Chem 2008; 54:617.

[68] Olatidoye AG, Wu AH, Feng YJ, Waters D. Prognostic role of troponin T versus troponin I in unstable angina pectoris for cardiac events with meta-analysis comparing published studies. Am J Cardiol 1998; 81:1405.

[69] Heidenreich PA, Alloggiamento T, Melsop K, et al. The prognostic value of troponin in patients with non-ST elevation acute coronary syndromes: a meta-analysis. J Am Coll Cardiol 2001; 38:478.

[70] Heeschen C, Hamm CW, Goldmann B, et al. Troponin concentrations for stratification of patients with acute coronary syndromes in relation to therapeutic efficacy of tirofiban. PRISM Study Investigators. Platelet Receptor Inhibition in Ischemic Syndrome Management. Lancet 1999; 354:1757.

[71] James S, Armstrong P, Califf R, et al. Troponin T levels and risk of 30-day outcomes in patients with the acute coronary syndrome: prospective verification in the GUSTO-IV trial. Am J Med 2003; 115:178.

[72] Ohman EM, Armstrong PW, White HD, et al. Risk stratification with a point-of-care cardiac troponin T test in acute myocardial infarction. GUSTOIII Investigators. Global Use of Strategies To Open Occluded Coronary Arteries. Am J Cardiol 1999; 84:1281.

[73] Giannitsis E, Müller-Bardorff M, Lehrke S, et al. Admission troponin T level predicts clinical outcomes, TIMI flow, and myocardial tissue perfusion after primary percutaneous intervention for acute ST-segment elevation myocardial infarction. Circulation 2001; 104:630.

[74] Ottani F, Galvani M, Nicolini FA, et al. Elevated cardiac troponin levels predict the risk of adverse outcome in patients with acute coronary syndromes. Am Heart J 2000; 140:917.

[75] Morrow DA, Antman EM, Tanasijevic M, et al. Cardiac troponin I for stratification of early outcomes and the efficacy of enoxaparin in unstable angina: a TIMI-11B substudy. J Am Coll Cardiol 2000; 36:1812.

[76] Lindahl B, Venge P, Wallentin L. Relation between troponin T and the risk of subsequent cardiac events in unstable coronary artery disease. The FRISC study group. Circulation 1996; 93:1651.

[77] Antman EM, Tanasijevic MJ, Thompson B, et al. Cardiac-specific troponin I levels to predict the risk of mortality in patients with acute coronary syndromes. N Engl J Med 1996; 335:1342.

[78] Ohman EM, Armstrong PW, Christenson RH, et al. Cardiac troponin T levels for risk stratification in acute myocardial ischemia. GUSTO IIA Investigators. N Engl J Med 1996; 335:1333.

[79] Hamm CW, Goldmann BU, Heeschen C, et al. Emergency room triage of patients with acute chest pain by means of rapid testing for cardiac troponin T or troponin I. N Engl J Med 1997; 337:1648.

[80] Lindahl B, Diderholm E, Lagerqvist B, et al. Mechanisms behind the prognostic value of troponin T in unstable coronary artery disease: a FRISC II substudy. J Am Coll Cardiol 2001; 38:979.

[81] Heeschen C, Hamm CW, Bruemmer J, Simoons ML. Predictive value of C-reactive protein and troponin T in patients with unstable angina: a comparative analysis. CAPTURE Investigators. Chimeric c7E3 AntiPlatelet Therapy in Unstable angina REfractory to standard treatment trial. J Am Coll Cardiol 2000; 35:1535.

[82] Lindahl B, Toss H, Siegbahn A, et al. Markers of myocardial damage and inflammation in relation to long-term mortality in unstable coronary artery disease. FRISC Study Group. Fragmin during Instability in Coronary Artery Disease. N Engl J Med 2000; 343:1139.

[83] Antman EM, Cohen M, Bernink PJ, et al. The TIMI risk score for unstable angina/non-ST elevation MI: A method for prognostication and therapeutic decision making. JAMA 2000; 284:835.

[84] Morrow DA, Cannon CP, Rifai N, et al. Ability of minor elevations of troponins I and T to predict benefit from an early invasive strategy in patients with unstable angina and non-ST elevation myocardial infarction: results from a randomized trial. JAMA 2001; 286:2405.

[85] Kleiman NS, Lakkis N, Cannon CP, et al. Prospective analysis of creatine kinase muscle-brain fraction and comparison with troponin T to predict cardiac risk and benefit of an invasive strategy in patients with non-ST-elevation acute coronary syndromes. J Am Coll Cardiol 2002; 40:1044.

[86] Diderholm E, Andrén B, Frostfeldt G, et al. The prognostic and therapeutic implications of increased troponin T levels and ST depression in unstable coronary artery disease: the FRISC II invasive troponin T electrocardiogram substudy. Am Heart J 2002; 143:760.

[87] Heeschen C, van Den Brand MJ, Hamm CW, Simoons ML. Angiographic findings in patients with refractory unstable angina according to troponin T status. Circulation 1999; 100:1509.

[88] Martinez MW, Babuin L, Syed IS, et al. Myocardial infarction with normal coronary arteries: a role for MRI? Clin Chem 2007; 53:995.

[89] Christiansen JP, Edwards C, Sinclair T, et al. Detection of myocardial scar by contrast-enhanced cardiac magnetic resonance imaging in patients with troponin-positive chest pain and minimal angiographic coronary artery disease. Am J Cardiol 2006; 97:768.

[90] Dokainish H, Pillai M, Murphy SA, et al. Prognostic implications of elevated troponin in patients with suspected acute coronary syndrome but no critical epicardial coronary disease: a TACTICS-TIMI-18 substudy. J Am Coll Cardiol 2005; 45:19.

[91] James SK, Armstrong P, Barnathan E, et al. Troponin and C-reactive protein have different relations to subsequent mortality and myocardial infarction after acute coronary syndrome: a GUSTO-IV substudy. J Am Coll Cardiol 2003; 41:916.

[92] Kontos MC, Shah R, Fritz LM, et al. Implication of different cardiac troponin I levels for clinical outcomes and prognosis of acute chest pain patients. J Am Coll Cardiol 2004; 43:958.

[93] Mueller C, Neumann FJ, Perruchoud AP, et al. Prognostic value of quantitative troponin T measurements in unstable angina/non-ST-segment elevation acute myocardial infarction treated early and predominantly with percutaneous coronary intervention. Am J Med 2004; 117:897.

[94] Newby LK, Christenson RH, Ohman EM, et al. Value of serial troponin T measures for early and late risk stratification in patients with acute coronary syndromes. The GUSTO-IIa Investigators. Circulation 1998; 98:1853.

[95] Antman EM. Troponin measurements in ischemic heart disease: more than just a black and white picture. J Am Coll Cardiol 2001; 38:987.

[96] Bessman SP, Carpenter CL. The creatine-creatine phosphate energy shuttle. Annu Rev Biochem 1985; 54:831.

[97] Roberts R, Gowda KS, Ludbrook PA, Sobel BE. Specificity of elevated serum MB creatine phosphokinase activity in the diagnosis of acute myocardial infarction. Am J Cardiol 1975; 36:433.

[98] Tsung JS, Tsung SS. Creatine kinase isoenzymes in extracts of various human skeletal muscles. Clin Chem 1986; 32:1568.

[99] Neumeier, D. Tissue specific and subcellular distribution of creatine kinase isoenzymes. In: Creatine Kinase Isoenzymes, Lang, H (Ed), Springer-Verlag, Berlin/Heidelberg 1981. p.85.

[100] Trask RV, Billadello JJ. Tissue-specific distribution and developmental regulation of M and B creatine kinase mRNAs. Biochim Biophys Acta 1990; 1049:182.

[101] Fontanet HL, Trask RV, Haas RC, et al. Regulation of expression of M, B, and mitochondrial creatine kinase mRNAs in the left ventricle after pressure overload in rats. Circ Res 1991; 68:1007.

[102] Wolf PL. Abnormalities in serum enzymes in skeletal muscle diseases. Am J Clin Pathol 1991; 95:293.

[103] Siegel AJ, Silverman LM, Evans WJ. Elevated skeletal muscle creatine kinase MB isoenzyme levels in marathon runners. JAMA 1983; 250:2835.

[104] Clark GL, Robison AK, Gnepp DR, et al. Effects of lymphatic transport of enzyme on plasma creatine kinase time-activity curves after myocardial infarction in dogs. Circ Res 1978; 43:162.

[105] Vatner SF, Baig H, Manders WT, Maroko PR. Effects of coronary artery reperfusion on myocardial infarct size calculated from creatine kinase. J Clin Invest 1978; 61:1048.

[106] Dillon MC, Calbreath DF, Dixon AM, et al. Diagnostic problem in acute myocardial infarction: CK-MB in the absence of abnormally elevated total creatine kinase levels. Arch Intern Med 1982; 142:33.

[107] Heller GV, Blaustein AS, Wei JY. Implications of increased myocardial isoenzyme level in the presence of normal serum creatine kinase activity. Am J Cardiol 1983; 51:24.

[108] Yusuf S, Collins R, Lin L, et al. Significance of elevated MB isoenzyme with normal creatine kinase in acute myocardial infarction. Am J Cardiol 1987; 59:245.

[109] Puleo PR, Guadagno PA, Roberts R, et al. Early diagnosis of acute myocardial infarction based on assay for subforms of creatine kinase-MB. Circulation 1990; 82:759.

[110] Puleo PR, Meyer D, Wathen C, et al. Use of a rapid assay of subforms of creatine kinase-MB to diagnose or rule out acute myocardial infarction. N Engl J Med 1994; 331:561.

[111] Jaffe AS, Landt Y, Parvin CA, et al. Comparative sensitivity of cardiac troponin I and lactate dehydrogenase isoenzymes for diagnosing acute myocardial infarction. Clin Chem 1996; 42:1770.

[112] Adams JE 3rd, Dávila-Román VG, Bessey PQ, et al. Improved detection of cardiac contusion with cardiac troponin I. Am Heart J 1996; 131:308.

[113] Adams JE 3rd, Sicard GA, Allen BT, et al. Diagnosis of perioperative myocardial infarction with measurement of cardiac troponin I. N Engl J Med 1994; 330:670.

[114] Larca LJ, Coppola JT, Honig S. Creatine kinase MB isoenzyme in dermatomyositis: a noncardiac source. Ann Intern Med 1981; 94:341.

[115] Lenke LG, Bridwell KH, Jaffe AS. Increase in creatine kinase MB isoenzyme levels after spinal surgery. J Spinal Disord 1994; 7:70.

[116] Badsha H, Gunes B, Grossman J, Brahn E. Troponin I Assessment of Cardiac Involvement in Patients With Connective Tissue Disease and an Elevated Creatine Kinase MB Isoform Report of Four Cases and Review of the Literature. J Clin Rheumatol 1997; 3:131.

[117] Hochberg MC, Koppes GM, Edwards CQ, et al. Hypothyroidism presenting as a polymyositis-like syndrome. Report of two cases. Arthritis Rheum 1976; 19:1363.

[118] Jaffe AS, Ritter C, Meltzer V, et al. Unmasking artifactual increases in creatine kinase isoenzymes in patients with renal failure. J Lab Clin Med 1984; 104:193.

[119] Gutovitz AL, Sobel BE, Roberts R. Progressive nature of myocardial injury in selected patients with cardiogenic shock. Am J Cardiol 1978; 41:469.

[120] Alexander JH, Sparapani RA, Mahaffey KW, et al. Association between minor elevations of creatine kinase-MB level and mortality in patients with acute coronary syndromes without ST-segment elevation. PURSUIT Steering Committee. Platelet Glycoprotein IIb/IIIa in Unstable Angina: Receptor Suppression Using Integrilin Therapy. JAMA 2000; 283:347.

[121] Savonitto S, Granger CB, Ardissino D, et al. The prognostic value of creatine kinase elevations extends across the whole spectrum of acute coronary syndromes. J Am Coll Cardiol 2002; 39:22.

[122] Halkin A, Stone GW, Grines CL, et al. Prognostic implications of creatine kinase elevation after primary percutaneous coronary intervention for acute myocardial infarction. J Am Coll Cardiol 2006; 47:951.

[123] Galla JM, Mahaffey KW, Sapp SK, et al. Elevated creatine kinase-MB with normal creatine kinase predicts worse outcomes in patients with acute coronary syndromes: results from 4 large clinical trials. Am Heart J 2006; 151:16.

[124] Lloyd-Jones DM, Camargo CA Jr, Giugliano RP, et al. Characteristics and prognosis of patients with suspected acute myocardial infarction and elevated MB relative index but normal total creatine kinase. Am J Cardiol 1999; 84:957.

[125] Newby LK, Roe MT, Chen AY, et al. Frequency and clinical implications of discordant creatine kinase-MB and troponin measurements in acute coronary syndromes. J Am Coll Cardiol 2006; 47:312.

[126] Rao SV, Ohman EM, Granger CB, et al. Prognostic value of isolated troponin elevation across the spectrum of chest pain syndromes. Am J Cardiol 2003; 91:936.

[127] Goodman SG, Steg PG, Eagle KA, et al. The diagnostic and prognostic impact of the redefinition of acute myocardial infarction: lessons from the Global Registry of Acute Coronary Events (GRACE). Am Heart J 2006; 151:654.

[128] Califf RM, Abdelmeguid AE, Kuntz RE, et al. Myonecrosis after revascularization procedures. J Am Coll Cardiol 1998; 31:241.

[129] Tardiff BE, Califf RM, Tcheng JE, et al. Clinical outcomes after detection of elevated cardiac enzymes in patients undergoing percutaneous intervention. IMPACT-II Investigators. Integrilin (eptifibatide) to Minimize Platelet Aggregation and Coronary Thrombosis-II. J Am Coll Cardiol 1999; 33:88.

[130] Simoons ML, van den Brand M, Lincoff M, et al. Minimal myocardial damage during coronary intervention is associated with impaired outcome. Eur Heart J 1999; 20:1112.

[131] Cavallini C, Savonitto S, Violini R, et al. Impact of the elevation of biochemical markers of myocardial damage on long-term mortality after percutaneous coronary intervention: results of the CK-MB and PCI study. Eur Heart J 2005; 26:1494.

[132] Cantor WJ, Newby LK, Christenson RH, et al. Prognostic significance of elevated troponin I after percutaneous coronary intervention. J Am Coll Cardiol 2002; 39:1738.

[133] Kizer JR, Muttrej MR, Matthai WH, et al. Role of cardiac troponin T in the long-term risk stratification of patients undergoing percutaneous coronary intervention. Eur Heart J 2003; 24:1314.

[134] Nageh T, Sherwood RA, Harris BM, et al. Cardiac troponin T and I and creatine kinase-MB as markers of myocardial injury and predictors of outcome following percutaneous coronary intervention. Int J Cardiol 2003; 92:285.

[135] Kini AS, Lee P, Marmur JD, et al. Correlation of postpercutaneous coronary intervention creatine kinase-MB and troponin I elevation in predicting mid-term mortality. Am J Cardiol 2004; 93:18.

[136] Wu AH, Boden WE, McKay RG. Long-term follow-up of patients with increased cardiac troponin concentrations following percutaneous coronary intervention. Am J Cardiol 2002; 89:1300.

[137] Miller WL, Garratt KN, Burritt MF, et al. Baseline troponin level: key to understanding the importance of post-PCI troponin elevations. Eur Heart J 2006; 27:1061.

[138] Prasad A, Rihal CS, Lennon RJ, et al. Significance of periprocedural myonecrosis on outcomes following Percutaneous coronary intervention. Circ Cardiovasc Intervent 2008; 1:9.

[139] Pierpont GL, McFalls EO. Interpreting troponin elevations: do we need multiple diagnoses? Eur Heart J 2009; 30:135.

[140] Prasad A, Singh M, Lerman A, et al. Isolated elevation in troponin T after percutaneous coronary intervention is associated with higher long-term mortality. J Am Coll Cardiol 2006; 48:1765.

[141] Nienhuis MB, Ottervanger JP, Dikkeschei B, et al. Prognostic importance of troponin T and creatine kinase after elective angioplasty. Int J Cardiol 2007; 120:242.

[142] Kleiman NS. Measuring troponin elevation after percutaneous coronary intervention: ready for prime time? J Am Coll Cardiol 2006; 48:1771.

[143] Costa MA, Carere RG, Lichtenstein SV, et al. Incidence, predictors, and significance of abnormal cardiac enzyme rise in patients treated with bypass surgery in the arterial revascularization therapies study (ARTS). Circulation 2001; 104:2689.

[144] Brener SJ, Lytle BW, Schneider JP, et al. Association between CK-MB elevation after percutaneous or surgical revascularization and three-year mortality. J Am Coll Cardiol 2002; 40:1961.

[145] Januzzi JL, Lewandrowski K, MacGillivray TE, et al. A comparison of cardiac troponin T and creatine kinase-MB for patient evaluation after cardiac surgery. J Am Coll Cardiol 2002; 39:1518.

[146] Steuer J, Bjerner T, Duvernoy O, et al. Visualisation and quantification of perioperative myocardial infarction after coronary artery bypass surgery with contrast-enhanced magnetic resonance imaging. Eur Heart J 2004; 25:1293.

[147] Carrier M, Pellerin M, Perrault LP, et al. Troponin levels in patients with myocardial infarction after coronary artery bypass grafting. Ann Thorac Surg 2000; 69:435.

[148] Croal BL, Hillis GS, Gibson PH, et al. Relationship between postoperative cardiac troponin I levels and outcome of cardiac surgery. Circulation 2006; 114:1468.

[149] Thielmann M, Massoudy P, Jaeger BR, et al. Emergency re-revascularization with percutaneous coronary intervention, reoperation, or conservative treatment in patients with acute perioperative graft failure following coronary artery bypass surgery. Eur J Cardiothorac Surg 2006; 30:117.

[150] Morrow DA, Cannon CP, Jesse RL, et al. National Academy of Clinical Biochemistry Laboratory Medicine Practice Guidelines: clinical characteristics and utilization of biochemical markers in acute coronary syndromes. Clin Chem 2007; 53:552.

4

Measurement of Myocardial Contractility in the Ischemic Heart – A Disease Immanent Uncertainty

Jens Broscheit
Department of Anethesiology, University Clinics of Würzburg
Germany

1. Introduction

The present compilation of scientific publications deals with the evaluation of a parameter of myocardial contractility (E'_{es}); the parameter can be exclusively measured using ultrasound, i.e. noninvasive and can be used for a load-independent quantification of myocardial contractility.

The standard procedure for measuring left ventricular (LV) contractility is by use of a conductance catheter with which LV volume and LV pressure can be determined simultaneously. In 1973, Sagawa (1) was the first to use this catheter, which had been developed at the University Hospital Leiden, and he was able to show that an elastance curve can be determined from a series of loop diagrams which were obtained under acute preload reduction. The slope of the elastance curve (E_{es}) increased when the positive inotropic substance isoprenaline was administered (Fig. 1).

For clinical use, however, the catheter is a monitoring procedure which is too invasive and thus involves too many risks; in the past few years there have been considerations to replace this procedure with one that is less invasive.

In 1994, Gorscan (2) presented a study with which he was able to show that LV volume can be estimated by continuous echocardiographic determination of the cross-sectional LV area and in 1997 Deanault from the same working group (3) showed that LV pressure can be approximated with the pressure from the radial artery. They generated a loop diagram from these surrogate parameters with which they could estimate LV contractility. In the years 2001-2003 the mathematicians Danielsen, Ottesen and Paladino (4-6) from the University of Roskilde published a model equation from which we deduce that, with simplified assumptions, the Doppler sonographic arterial flow would have to change in proportion to pressure and we asked ourselves if contractility could also be estimated with a flow-area relationship.

2. Question

The thoughts presented here are a model for measuring LV contractility as it could be determined in the patient, i.e. exclusively based on ultrasound and thus not very invasive.

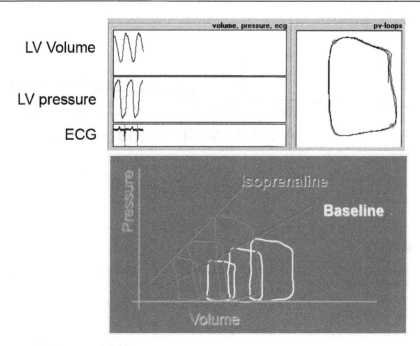

Sagawa K, et al. Am J Cardiol 1977; 40:748-753

Fig. 1. Determination of the properties of elastance curves

This raises the question of whether contractility can in fact be estimated using the index E'_{es}, which has been deduced from this theoretical model.

If the elastance of the flow-area relationship is exclusively considered as a surrogate parameter to estimate myocardial contractility in the classical sense, then E'_{es} is not a new parameter. If it is assumed, however, that the elastance of the flow-area relationship is based on a completely new mathematical model, i.e. that of the mathematicians Danielsen, Ottesen and Paladino, then we are possibly dealing with a new parameter and deviations between the classical parameter E_{es} and E'_{es} are then starting points for new examinations.

3. Background

Ultrasound-based determination of myocardial contractility: theoretical principles

The ability to actively shorten the cardiac muscle, i.e. of contractility, of the left ventricle is based on a complex process (7,8) during which individual mechanisms have to follow one another precisely. Muscle contraction is based on mechanisms and interactions associated with muscle proteins, enzymes, ions and energy sources. The large-scale structure, as well as the small-scale structure of the muscle, are involved in the contractility of the hollow muscular organ which forms the left chamber of the heart or left ventricle. Apart from power transmission towards contraction, the prevention or diversion of shearing forces is an important task which the muscle carries out through mechanisms of mechanical connections, but also through mechanisms of regulation by synchronizing the contraction of the muscle fibers.

First attempts to describe the contractility of a hollow muscular organ from a mechanical point of view date back to Otto Frank in 1985 (9). Frank determined the pressure of the individual end-diastolic volumes by conducting experiments with a single chamber frog heart as well as the maximum pressure recruitable from this relaxation period (isovolumeric maximum) and the maximum ejection fraction (isotonic or isobaric maximum). The curves established from this resulted in a pressure-volume diagram in which the maximums to be achieved from the relaxation period were connected through the contraction curve (2). Otto Frank deduced the cardiac cycle from this:

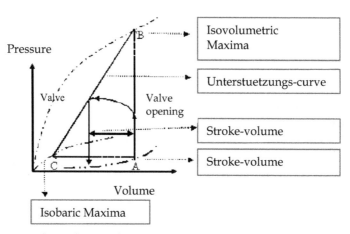

Fig. 2. LV pressure-volume diagram by Otto Frank.

The ventricle is filled with volume (preload) and during the process internal pressure in the chamber increases. Then the pressure in the chamber increases through contraction along the isometric maximum against the closed valve until the valve opens which, during the relaxation phase (diastole), prevents reflux from the aorta into the ventricle. While the heart is pumping out volume against the arterial load (afterload), it is pumping in the sense of an auxotonic contraction; this leads to a further increase of arterial pressure and to a decrease in volume through ejection in the ventricle. During the following relaxation phase the pressure in the ventricle decreases to reach its resting level and the chamber is filled again. The cardiac cycle can thus be described through a pressure-volume relationship which is known as the "work diagram" in literature.

In later experiments, Starling (10) deduced the s-shaped connection between the surface of the work diagram and the necessary preload. The two main differences between the concept described by Otto Frank and the one developed by Starling are that the contraction of the left ventricle cannot only be described as a function of filling or preload, but also as a function of time. Another difference is that when it comes to measurements, the left ventricular function is always determined in connection with the arterial vascular system behind it.

In 1959, Warner deduced the calculation of ventricular compliance C from the correlation described by Frank by relating volume V_v and the corresponding pressure P_v at the end of diastole and at the end of systole

$$C = \frac{V_v}{P_v}$$

and thus created a constant. From this formal approach, two different mathematical terms for the description of LV contraction can be concluded. In 1961, Seelen (11) described contraction through fixed capacitive reactance in series with pressure varying depending on time and in 1973, Suga (1) defined ventricular elastance $E(t)$ through an inverse function of the compliance $C(t)$ function.

$$E(t) = \frac{P_v(t)}{V_v(t) - V_d}$$

with the SI-unit [$m^{-4} \cdot kg \cdot s^{-2}$], while V_d represents constant, diastolic volume. The index (t) in this case means that the end-systolic point was determined using an iterative method in which the same loop is crossed by a tangent several times and with varying time (time-varying elastance). In the experimental determination of $E(t)$, the same problems arise as in the correlation already developed by Starling. The index $E(t)$ cannot be determined separately from the vascular system and it is not a function of time.

To get around these problems, Beneken 1965 (12) developed a closed-loop model of the cardiovascular system, which was based on the work of Liljestrand 1938 (13) and Hill 1922 (14), and in which contraction of the heart is calculated through the contractile element described by Hill, embedded in a three-element windkessel model. Further geometrical adjustments yielded an n-element model, which was mathematically described with the finite-element method.

Based on the evaluation described by Hill, Danielsen (4) later developed a model which differentiated between an isovolumetric ventricle and an ejecting left ventricle under arterial load. In the latter model, the direct proportional correlation between arterial pressure P_a and LV outflow Q_v was deduced as follows:

$$\dot{P}_s = -\frac{1}{R_s C_s} P_s + \frac{1}{C_s} Q_v,$$

with R_s as a global peripheral resistance, R_0 as characteristic aortic impedance, C_s as total arterial compliance, P_s as systolic pressure and P_s as the change of arterial pressure with time. This equation can be transformed to This equation can be transformed to:

$$\dot{Q}_v = -\frac{1}{L_v} P_s - \frac{R_0}{L_v} Q_v + \frac{1}{L_v} P_v(t, V),$$

with L_v as inductance directly above the aortic valve and Q_v as a change of flow with time. With the simplified assumption that L_v is constant, the above equation can be simplified as follows.

$$P_a = P_s + R_0 Q_v$$

With the assumption that R_0 is constant and P_a changes in direct proportion to P_s the equation is:

$$P_a \approx Q_v$$

Olufsen (15) showed in his one-dimensional dynamic model of the systemic arteries that, corresponding to the Navier-Stokes equation, pressure changes directly proportional to flow in large vessels such as the arteria carotis communis. The model-based experimental examinations confirm that the flow generated through the left ventricle is the connecting link between the heart and vessel blood system.

Against this backdrop, our work group had the idea of developing an index $E'_{es,}$, analogous to $E(t)$, based on the iteratively determined end-systolic points on the work diagram. This index E'_{es} was to be determined by $V_d(t)$ and blood flow $V_v(t)$ of an artery in proximity to the heart:

$$E'_{es} = \frac{V_v(t)}{V_v(t) - V_d}$$

with the SI unit [s-1]. The ventricular volume, measured during several cardiac cycles, can be determined using ultrasound technology by estimating it with the help of the surface A in the transgastral short-axis-view. Blood flow Q can be estimated through the blood flow velocity F in the arteria carotis communis measured with the Doppler technology. This then yields the following equation:

$$E'_{es} = \frac{F_v(t)}{A_v(t) - A_d}$$

The deduced index E'_{es} displays the following important differences compared to the index E_{es} :

1. By implementing blood flow velocity, the index becomes a function of time.
2. By measuring blood flow velocity in a large artery, the index becomes connected to the vascular system.
3. Through the measuring method used, the index E'_{es} can be completely determined in a noninvasive way, as both F and A are ultrasound parameters.

Measuring methods used

The measuring methods used in this context are conductance and ultrasound methods. Using these methods, myocardial contractility was measured.

Conductance catheter method

A conductance catheter was used for the simultaneous recording of LV pressure and the volume signal (16). The catheter consists of pressure-conductivity transducers. While the blood pressure signal was mechanically measured at the tip of the catheter using a pressure transducer and was subsequently transformed into electric impulses, determination of volume is carried out electromagnetically by measuring the conductivity of the surrounding compartments. The catheter consists of four electrodes and one pressure sensor. The electrodes are fitted below the pressure sensor in pairs. The measurement of cardiac blood volumes using these electrodes is based on an electric field which is established through the outer electrodes in the left ventricle. Two potential differences at the inner electrodes are continuously recorded to measure the conductance between the electrodes in the ventricle.

With the formula

$$V_i(t) = \frac{1}{\alpha} \bullet \rho L_{a^2}(G_i(t) - G_{pi})$$

intraventricular volume V(t) is calculated. With a being a volume calibration factor, p being the electric resistance of blood, L being the distance between the electrodes, G_i describing the overall conductance and G_{pi} describing the conductance of the surrounding tissue; this conductance is called "parallel conductance". This calculation makes a continuous and in vivo recording of volumes in real-time possible.

Ultrasound method

Using the ultrasound-Doppler method, the flow velocity of erythrocytes can be measured with the help of the Doppler effect. The Doppler effect arises because echoes reflected by the erythrocytes have higher or lower frequencies than the signals sent out, depending on the flow velocity and flow direction. The differences in frequency are implemented electronically in readable and recordable curves. In the continuous-wave Doppler (CW Doppler) technique, which is used for detection, one transmitter and one receiver work simultaneously and continuously in the transducer. By mixing it with suitable high frequency signals and with electronic filters, the spectrum of the Doppler frequencies or velocities and the direction can be determined from the returning wave in the evaluation electronics. The disadvantage of this method is that it is not possible to determine the base range of the Doppler echo; however, even relatively high velocities can be recorded.

With the two-dimensional, light-modulated presentation of the echoes, an immediately visible, animated picture is generated through energy and intensity proportional light points that vary according to brightness and as a result of a scan carried out in two directions and in layers. Tissue structures become visible because the points that are represented in shades of gray in relation to the intensity of the echo - as far as they originate from comparable structures - flow together to form areas and lines. The semi-automatic detection of contours serves to detect endocardial interfaces within the "region of interest" (ROI). Semi-automatic contour tracking is based on a seeded ROI algorithm which combines all adjacent pixels within a user-defined signal intensity area. The selected (seed) pixel is the starting point. In automatic segmentation, a small ROI can be positioned in the area of interest. The signal intensity area important for the growth algorithm is automatically taken from the ROI statistics (minimum to maximum value). The area defined in this way can be corrected interactively. For an ROI correction, the boundaries are activated by a click of the mouse. These boundaries can also be corrected interactively. After having selected the acoustic windows relevant for the approximation of volume - transgastral short-axis-view of the left ventricle - the window setting at an end-diastolic phase image was adjusted to achieve an ideal contrast for the detection of endocardial boundaries. This window setting as well as the curves of the ventricular area presented in the ultrasound image were then checked in all phase images of the cardiac cycle. This setting was used for the following examinations.

Measuring parameters

End-systolic elastance is derived from the end-systolic pressure-volume relation (ESPVR). The elastance model was introduced by Sagawa and Suga. (17). Using isolated rabbit hearts, they made the observation that the end-systolic pressure volume coordinates move along a straight line in the case of acute preload reduction. This could also be observed when acute preload reduction occurred at different levels of dilatation of the left ventricle (Fig. 1) is it a picture legend? A difference is made between two elastances: time-dependent elastance E_{max} and time-varying elastance E_{es}.

In this model, E_{max} describes the slope of the end-systolic linear regression curves.

In this context the time-dependent elastance $E(t)$ from the equation

$$E(t) = \frac{P(t)}{V(t) - VL(t)}$$

is determined, with $P(t)$ = instantaneous intraventricular pressure; $V(t)$ = instantaneous intraventricular volume; $V0$ = volume, if $P(t) = 0$. E_{es} is elastance at the point in time when $E(t)$ reaches its maximum, i.e. when active contraction is at its maximum. E_{es} is calculated from the slope of the linear regression curves, which is time-varying and results from the maximum of the points.

$$\frac{P}{V - V_0}$$

The calculation of maximum is repeated several times through fixed point iteration until the slope of the line is constant. E_{es} is determined if, in case of fluctuations in afterload, the time in which the end-systolic state is reached fluctuates and consequently ESPVR does not exactly meet the angle of the loop diagram and E_{max} is calculated from points which lie ahead of the end-systolic one. E_{max} is then steeper than E_{es}. While E_{max} is the basis for models concerning the mathematical adjustment of the left ventricular function, E_{es} is used for the experimental quantification of LV contractility. The calculation formula for the indices E_{max} and E_{es} is not presented in a consistent manner in literature, however. The index E'_{es} was determined analogous to the index Ees, with the difference that the flow-volume diagram was the basis for calculation

A positive inotropic effect, induced through dobutamine, can be observed through an increase of E_{es}, i.e. an increase in the slope of the linear regression curves. The opposite occurs in decreasing inotropy, when it is triggered by a β- receptor blocker like esmolol (Fig. 1) is it a picture legend?, for instance.

Hemodynamic interventions

The main goal of the studies were the controlled, targeted and pathophysiological interventions with sequential application of dobutamine, esmolol, akrinor, hydroxyethyl starch and sodium nitroprusside, with which the degree of correspondence of the two measuring methods was determined. The properties of these substances, which will be described in the following section, were the reason for them being used.

Modification of contractility through dobutamine and esmolol

Dobutamine has the effect of an α1-, β1- and β2-agonist, while β1 stimulation of the heart is the most immediate effect. The main effects of dobutamine result from this, i.e. the increase of contractility of the myocardial cells and a dosage-dependent marked increase in heart rate. This leads to increased stroke volume (SV) and cardiac output (CO). The substance has a short half-life period of approx. 2 minutes and is broken down in inactive metabolites. It is thus applied per continuitatem. needs spell check here – it is the latin spelling and ok!.

Esmolol has the effect of a β1-antagonist and is thus cardioselective at the myocardium. The main effects are a decrease in heart rate and the inhibition of contractility. This leads to a decrease in stroke volume and in cardiac output. The half-life period is only approx. 9 minutes, as esmolol, in contrast to other beta blockers, is not broken down in an organ-dependent way, but is metabolized by esterases hydrolases. For this reason, esmolol has to be administered in a continuous or repetitive way.

Modification of load through hydroxyethyl starch, akrinor and sodium nitroprusside

In statistics or kinematics, load is a unit of measurement for the force that works on a medium. Accordingly and as far as the left ventricle is concerned, preload is the force that results in the extension of fibers at the end of diastole or directly before systole and which is limited by the maximum resting length of the muscle fiber. Afterload is a force influencing the ventricle; this force counteracts ejection out of the ventricle into the cardiovascular system. In practice, preload is referred to as the end-diastolic volume in the heart. The fact that the standard index E_{es} is load-independent , i.e. that changes in preload and afterload of the left ventricle mostly do not change the contractility index over wide periods, is an important characteristic of this measurement. Changes in load induce changes in contraction force, contractility remains unchanged, however.

Hydroxyethyl starch is a synthetically produced polymer and, like dextrane, and gelatine is used for the substitution of intravascular volume. End-diastolic volume was thus increased.

Akrinor is a fixed combination of the two active ingredients cafedrin and theodrenaline. Blood pressure is primarily increased through an alpha-receptor-mediated, arterial vasoconstriction. Then contractility and heart rate are slightly increased through a less intense stimulation of beta receptors.

Apart from inhibiting guanylate cyclase and consecutively releasing nitric oxide in the smooth musculature of the vascular wall, sodium nitroprusside has a vasodilative effect on both at the resistance vessels of the arterial system and at the capacitance vessels of the venous system. Due to the short half-life period of less than 10 minutes, continuous administration is necessary.

4. Determination of preload recruitable stroke work and elastance by the relation of arterial blood flow velocity to left ventricular area

The question whether contractility can be estimated with a flow-area relationship was the starting point for this study.

In a first animal experiment, 8 Göttinger minipigs were studied in an open chest preparation. An arterial manometer was placed in the femoral artery and a microtip catheter for the measurement of LV pressure was advanced into the left ventricle from the apex. A flexible TEE probe was fixed on the myocardium to sonographically estimate volume with LV area measurement. Finally, the arteria carotis communis was dissected to fix a U-shaped 8-MHz CW Doppler probe on it. Then an inferior vena cava occlusion was performed to reduce preload. A central venous catheter was implanted for the pharmacological intervention. Via this catheter, contractility was sequentially increased by the administration of dobutamine, it was decreased by the administration of the beta-blocker esmolol and preload was significantly increased with a plasma expander. A software exclusively developed by the Institute of Experimental Physics was used for data acquisition as well as data presentation and analysis (Fig. 3). During the examination we began to realize that we were generating loop diagrams and could calculate elastance.

Feasibility study - Method

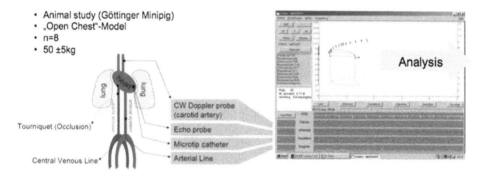

Determination of Preload-Recruitable Stroke Work and Elastance by the Relationship of Arterial Blood Flow Velocity to Left Ventricular Area*

- Animal study (Göttinger Minipig)
- „Open Chest"-Model
- n=8
- 50 ±5kg

Tourniquet (Occlusion)*

Central Venous Line*

CW Doppler probe (carotid artery)
Echo probe
Microtip catheter
Arterial Line

Analysis

Sequential intervention with
1. Dobutamin (5µg/kgKG, Inotrpy ↑)
2. Esmolol (0,5mg/kgKG, Inotropy ↓)
3. Plasmaexpander (10ml/kgKG, Preload↑)

*Broscheit J, Kessler M, et al. J Cardiothorac Vasc Anesth. 2004 Aug; 18(4): 415-22

Fig. 3. Diagram for the experiment set-up of the study "Determination of Preload Recruitable Stroke Work and Elastance by the Relation of Arterial Blood Flow Velocity to Left Ventricular Area".

The data in table 2 (3b) show that the change in contractility was reliably detected through the change of slope of the individual elastance curves. A change of preload through the plasma expander did not influence the slope of the elastance curves.

To sum up, this study showed that contractility can be estimated with parameters which are deduced from flow-area relationships.

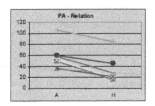 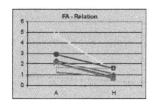 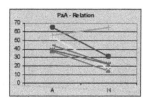

Abbreviations: PA – LVpressure vs. LVarea relation [mmHg/cm²]
                 FA – blood flow velocity vs. LVarea relation [cm/s/cm²]
                 PaA- art. rad vs. LVarea relation [mmHg/cm²]

	PA - Relation			FA - Relation			PaA- Relation		
	B	**E**	**Δ**	**B**	**E**	**Δ**	**B**	**E**	**Δ**
Mean	60.0	34.5	45.4*	2.4	1.2	45.3*	49.2	29.9	42.6 *
± SD	± 24.0	± 22.7	± 20.0	± 1.1	± 10.8	± 24.2	± 15.9	± 0.4	± 30.2

B = baseline, E = Esmolol 0.5 mg/kgBW,
Δ = increase of the slope in %, * =signtest p < 0,05

→ Inotropic changes can be detected by the flow-area relation

Fig. 3b. Feasibility study - Results

5. Time-varying elastance concept applied to the relation of carotid arterial flow velocity and left ventricular area

In the previous study, changes in inotropy could in fact be detected with the help of the flow-area relationship and the following study was to answer the question as to how this procedure corresponds to the standard procedure.

In an animal experiment, 25 Göttinger minipigs were studied in a closed chest preparation. After a puncture of the femoral artery, the conductance catheter was placed in the left ventricle under fluoroscopy. The cross-sectional LV area was determined in this study using a transthoracic probe and the arteria carotis communis was studied as before. A pulmonalis catheter was used for the calibration of the conductance catheter and a Forgarty catheter, which was advanced into the inferior vena cava, was used for preload reduction. The central venous catheter served as a line for the pharmacological interventions. Like in the previous study, contractility was sequentially increased by the administration of dobutamine, it was decreased by the administration of the beta-blocker esmolol and preload was significantly increased with a plasma expander. Additionally, afterload reduction was induced through akrinor.

For the collection and processing of data, software developed by Paul Steendijk from the experimental cardiology of the University Leiden was used in this study. Pressure volumes and flow-area relationships could be described using this software. The elastance of the LV pressure-volume relationship is referred to as E_{es} in literature and we called the elastance of the flow-area relationship E'_{es}.

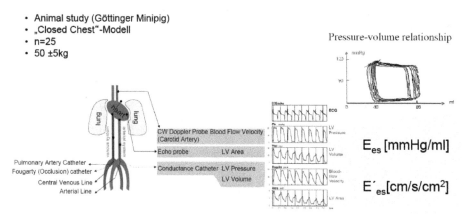

Fig. 4. Diagram for the experiment set-up of the study "Time-Varying Elastance Concept Applied to the Relation of Carotid Arterial Flow Velocity and Left Ventricular Area"

n = 25	Baseline	Dobutamine	Esmolol	Akrinor	Volume
HR (bpm)	64 ± 11	94 ± 32*	56 ± 7	64 ± 23	60 ± 19
E_{es} (mmHg/mL)	5.8 ± 3.04	10.1 ± 4.19*	3.7 ± 2.4*	8.31 ± 3.58	6.1 ± 2.8
E'_{es} (cm³/min)	0.68 ± 0.288	1.24 ± 0.458*	0.44 ± 0.15*	0.98 ± 0.379	0.69 ± 0.283

NOTE. All interventions were performed after complete reversal of hemodynamic changes to baseline. HR, heart rate; Ees, time-varying elastance; E´es, time-varying elastance of velocity; LV, area relation; *$p < 0.05$ versus baseline.

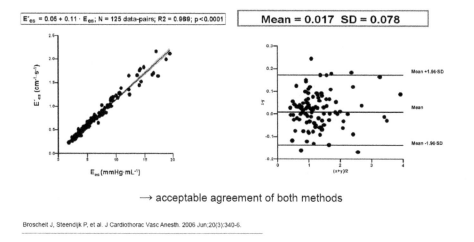

→ acceptable agreement of both methods

Broscheit J, Steendijk P, et al. J Cardiothorac Vasc Anesth. 2006 Jun;20(3):340-6.

Fig. 4b. Validational study (Conductance-Catheter) – Results

In relation to the initial values, the values obtained from both procedures displayed changes in inotropy. A regression analysis was carried out using the pooled data. A significant linear correlation between the two measuring methods became evident. The Blant-Altman analysis showed that both methods correspond to each other acceptably.

6. The relationship between carotid blood-flow velocity and left ventricular area during acute regional ischemia

This study was to answer the question as to how the two measuring methods would correspond to each other in the case of a myocardial wall motion abnormality.

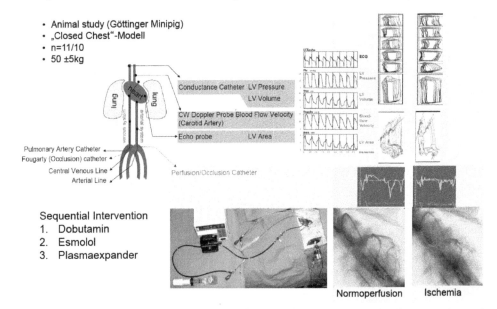

Fig. 5. Diagram for the experimental set-up of the study "The Relationship between Carotid Blood-flow Velocity and Left Ventricular Area during Acute Regional Ischemia".

In an animal experiment, 11 Göttinger minipigs were studied in a closed chest preparation. We advanced a coronary occlusion-perfusion catheter into the ramus circumflexus of the left coronary artery from the arteria femoralis. This catheter makes it possible to occlude a coronary artery while at the same time perfusing it with arterial blood using an adjustable roller pump. Standardized reduction of myocardial wall motion in the circulation area of the coronary artery was monitored by determining the systolic, radial strain rate. The strain rate is the rate of myocardial deformation and thus a unit of measurement for myocardial function. As the arteria femoralis was being used by the catheter, we advanced the conductance catheter through the right arteria carotis communis. Apart from that, preparation was the same as in the previous study.

Fig. 4 shows the loop diagram under normal perfusion and under ischemic conditions. The segmental loops of the conductance catheter deform under ischemia in the corresponding areas. This deformation was used for the calculation of an internal flow fraction, which arises when myocardial contraction cannot be completely transformed into an arterial flow.

	Baseline	Dobutamine	Esmolol	Ringer's Lactate	Perfusion State
E_{es} (mmHg/mL)	6.9 ± 2.7	12.8 ± 5.4*	4.4 ± 1.7*	6.4 ± 2.3	Normal
E_{es} (mmHg/ mL)	7.7 ± 4.2	11.8 ± 5.9*	4.9 ± 2.6*	5.0 ± 1.5	Ischemic
E'_{es} (mL/s/cm²)	0.54 ± 0.18	1.15 ± 0.42*	0.38 ± 0.14*	0.56 ± 0.13	Normal
E' (ml /s/cm²)	0.59 ± 0.12	0.88 ± 0.33*	0.77 ± 0.15*	0.41 ± 0.11*†	Ischemic
IFF_{sys} (%)	10 ± 17.7	12 ± 14	11 ± 8.9	21 ± 12.9	Normal
IFF_{sys} (%)	37 ± 24.7†	27 ± 24.6	35 ± 20.7†	21 ± 12.9*	Ischemic

NOTE. Normal perfused myocardium n=11; ischemic conditions, n=10. Abbreviations: Ees, end-systolic elastance calculated from the pressure-volume relation; E=es, end-systolic elastance calculated from the flow-area relation; IFFsys, systolic internal flow fraction. *Significance versus corresponding baseline value ($p<0.05$), †Significance versus corresponding nonischemic value ($p<0.05$).

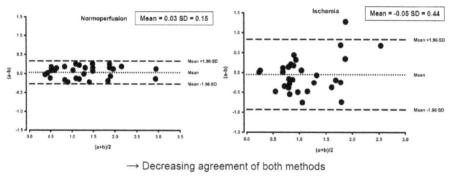

→ Decreasing agreement of both methods

Broscheit J, Weidemann F, Strotmann J, et al. J Cardiothorac Vasc Anesth. 2008 Dec;22(6):823-31.

Fig. 5b. Validational study during regional ischemia - Results

As the graph is directly taken from another journal, please get the copyright. I do realize that the author for this chapter is also the author for that article. However, the copyright need to be obtained as a formality from the journal. Table 1 (III 5b) shows that both procedures, independent of myocardial perfusion, could detect changes in inotropy. What stands out, however, is that the application of a plasma expander under myocardial ischemia leads to significant changes of the slope of the flow-area relationship compared to the initial values. The internal flow fraction also changed significantly under these conditions. Regression analysis in Fig. 5 (do you mean 5b? 5 is not a statistical analysis under ischemic conditions showed a decrease in the regression coefficient, linear correlation remained significant, however. The Bland-Alman analysis in Fig. 6 showed that the correspondence of the two parameters decreases.

The results of the study carried out showed that a valid assessment of myocardial contractility is possible with the flow-area relationship. Myocardial wall motion abnormalities constitute a limitation of the procedure.

7. Dobutamine induces ineffective work in regional ischaemic myocardium: An experimental strain rate imaging study

This study is to answer the question as to whether the results of the previous study can also be reflected by parameters of regional contractility.

In an animal experiment, 11 Göttinger minipigs were studied in a closed chest preparation. We advanced a coronary occlusion-perfusion catheter into the ramus circumflexus of the left coronary artery from the arteria femoralis. This catheter makes it possible to occlude a coronary artery while at the same time perfusing it with arterial blood using an adjustable roller pump. Standardized reduction of myocardial wall motion in the circulation area of the coronary artery was monitored by determining the strain rate. Apart from that, radial strain of the myocardium during systole was also determined. Strain is a unit of measurement for myocardial deformation. As the arteria femoralis was occupied by the catheter, we advanced the conductance catheter through the right arteria carotis communis.

The results show that a decrease of radial strain in the ischemic region can be documented under regional ischemia. Parallel to this, regional ischemia led to an increase in radial strain in the non ischemic myocardium. The stimulation of contractility with dobutamine intensifies the effect.

The present results confirm those of the previous study, i.e. that regional ischemia of the myocardium of 30% does not lead to a decrease of global contractility because contractility of the myocardium of the non-ischemic region is increased in a compensatory way. The increase of internal flow fraction is based on this effect, as has been shown in the previous study.

8. The relationship between carotid arterial flow and the left ventricular area is valid to indicate contractility in states of cerebral autoregulation and decreased arterial pressure

The present study is based on the question as to whether both measuring methods correspond under the condition of an arterial hypotension. Hypotension can activate mechanisms which, independent of systemic blood pressure, ensure constant blood flow in important organs such as the heart. To determine the flow-area relationship, we measure flow velocity in large vessels which supply the brain with blood; for this reason these mechanisms could have an effect on the flow-area relationship.

In an animal experiment, we studied 9 merino sheep and measured cortical microperfusion (flux) with the laser Doppler and we also determined tissue oxygen partial pressure ($p_{(ti)}O_2$) and tissue metabolism through microdialysis. We proceeded as in a validation study, the difference being that we fixed the TEE probe onto the myocardium with a minithoracotomy.

Arterial blood pressure was, on the one hand, decreased by esmolol and on the other hand by the pure vasodilator sodium nitroprusside. Both pharmaceuticals were dosed in such a way that a mean arterial pressure of 50mmHg could be maintained for 20 minutes.

The table shows that the hypotension triggered by sodium nitroprusside did not lead to any other changes of the circulatory system and of the cortical and myocardial parameters. The hypotension triggered by esmolol, however, led to a decrease in cardiac output and to an increase in LV end-diastolic pressure. This was associated with a decrease in cortical microcirculation as well as with a decrease in tissue oxygen partial pressure. During the decrease in tissue oxygen partial pressure, the metabolites of the anaerobic metabolism increased. Furthermore an increase in internal flow fraction (IFF_{sys}) could be observed, indicating myocardial wall motion abnormalities. The hypotension triggered by esmolol led to a critical decrease of oxygen being supplied to the cortex and to the myocardium.

As in the previous studies, a linear correlation between flow-area relationship and LV pressure could be detected under the influence of sodium nitroprusside. The correlation between the two relationships was acceptable as the Bland-Altman analysis shows. The decrease of contractility induced by esmolol was also detected through the flow-area relationship. But the degree of correlation and the degree of correspondence of both parameters decreased significantly. This decrease probably results from an increase of the internal flow fraction as an indication of myocardial wall motion abnormalities. This correlation could already be detected in the previous studies. It remains unclear, however, which hemodynamic constellation led to the wall motion abnormalities – the increase in end-diastolic volume and/ or the decrease of cardiac output. Both parameters determine myocardial perfusion.

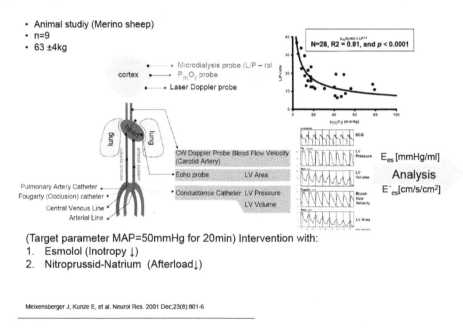

(Target parameter MAP=50mmHg for 20min) Intervention with:
1. Esmolol (Inotropy ↓)
2. Nitroprussid-Natrium (Afterload↓)

Meixensberger J, Kunze E, et al. Neurol Res. 2001 Dec;23(8):801-6

Fig. 6. Diagram for the experiment set-up of the study "The Relationship between Carotid Arterial Flow and the Left Ventricular Area is valid to indicate contractility in states of cerebral autoregulation and decreased arterial pressure

An increase in end-diastolic volume is connected with an increase in left ventricular radius. According to the law of Laplace, the increase in radius is tantamount to an increase in myocardial wall tension in diastole. During diastole the myocardium is perfused an increase in wall tension can lead to a decrease of coronary blood flow which means that oxygen supply is higher than oxygen demand. In this context, myocardial wall motion abnormalities can occur as an indication of hypoperfusion. A decrease in cardiac output is directly connected to a decrease of oxygen supply to all organs, i.e. also to the myocardium, which can result in insufficient oxygen supply.

The results of the study carried out showed that a valid assessment of myocardial contractility is possible with the flow-area relationship.

	Baseline	SNP	Esmolol
MAP [mmHg]	90 ±16	60 ±1*	48 ±6*
E$_{es}$ [mmHg cm^{-3}]	3.0 ±0.9	3.0 ±0.7	1.0 ±0.2*+
E'$_{es}$ [cm^{-3}]	0.89 ±0.24	0.76 ±0.27	0.36 ±0.21*+
Flux [mm·s^{-1}]	1	0.84 ±0.20	0.63 ±0.30*
p$_{ti}$O$_2$ [mmHg]	33 ±23	34 ±7	14 ±13*+
L/P-ratio [-]	12 ±3	19 ±8	26 ±15*+

NOTE: Mean ± standard deviation; n = 9.

Abbreviations: Ees, endsystolic elastance; E'es end-systolic elastance of the flow velocity-area relationship; Flux – cortical microcirculation; L/P-ratio, ratio of cortical lactate and pyruvate values; MAP, mean arterial pressure; p(ti)O2, cortical partial oxygen pressure in the tissue; SNP, sodium nitroprusside. # p < 0.05 compared with baseline. + p < 0.05 compared with SNP.

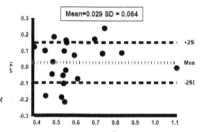

Bland-Altman analysis showing the limits of agreement and bias comparing conductance catheter derived Ees and ultrasonic based E'es. The limits of agreement (1.96 SD) were 0.13

⟶ acceptable agreement of both methods

Broschelt J, Kunze E, et al. I J Anesthesiology. 2008 Jan;18 (1):1-16

Fig. 6b. Validational study during arterial hypotension - Results

9. Association of increased myocardial contractility and elevated end-diastolic wall tension with short-term myocardial ischemia: A pressure-volume analysis

The present study is to answer the question whether myocardial hypoperfusion can be triggered by an LV hypervolemia, even if arterial pressure as well as cardiac output are in an "adequate" range - as literature usually calls it.

To answer this question, 15 Göttinger minipigs were studied in an open chest preparation. A catheter was placed in the arteria femoralis to measure pressure and a probe ,similar to those used for transoesophageal echocardiography, was fixed on the myocardium. A microtip catheter was inserted from the apex of the left ventricle for continuous pressure measurement. A catheter for microdialysis was implanted into the myocardium in the flow area of the left coronary artery. Finally, the arteria carotis communis was dissected to fix a U-shaped 8-MHz CW Doppler probe on it. A catheter in the femoral vein was used for pharmacological interventions.

Myocardial contractility was increased permanently through continuous application of dobutamine. A steady state was assumed after 20 minutes. Esmolol was administered in such a way that the heart rate - in relation to frequency - was lowered by at least 25% for 20 minutes under continuous infusion of dobutamin. Subsequently esmolol application was stopped so that dobutamin could again unfold its contractility-increasing effect. For comparison, only Esmolol was subsequently administered to another group - to the same amount as dobutamine and esmolol had been administered in the dobutamin-esmolol group. As expected, the table shows that when dobutamine and esmolol are administered at the same time, the heart rate decreases and contractility decreases later as well. Through the decrease in heart rate, LV volume increases in this phase and thus - according to the law of Laplace - diastolic myocardial wall tension increases as well. Dobutamine initially stimulates contractility but despite sufficient arterial pressure and cardiac output, oxygen supply is still lower than oxygen demand. Oxygen demand is then lowered by the decrease in contractility and the indications of hypoperfusion recede under identical wall tension. When the effect of esmolol starts to wear off, the contractility-stimulating effect of dobutamin comes back first and later the heart rate increases again. During this phase, increased wall tension leads to myocardial hypoperfusion again. Esmolol alone induces increased wall tension but no myocardial hypoperfusion.

The results of the present study show that an increase in myocardial wall tension alone is not necessarily associated with myocardial hypoperfusion. If, however, oxygen demand increases in this situation, or, as in the previous study, cardiac output and arterial pressure are reduced, the oxygen supply to the myocardium can sink below its oxygen demand. In this context, myocardial wall motion disorders can form as an indication of such an imbalance which in turn can lower the correlation of the two relations.

10. Conclusion and outlook

The results of the examination carried out allow the conclusion that a valid estimation of myocardial contractility is possible. Myocardial wall motion abnormalities limit the measuring accuracy of this new procedure. These myocardial wall motion abnormalities can occur if increased LV end-diastolic volume is associated with low cardiac output or an increased myocardial oxygen requirement.

In further investigations we would like to try to answer the question as to whether the acute afterload reduction necessary for the determination of elastance can also be induced through a Valsalva maneuver.

By using a 3-dimensional transoesophageal echocardiography, we would like to answer the question if measuring accuracy can possibly be significantly improved. On the one hand, using 3-dimensional echocardiography, similar to what is possible with a conductance catheter, could make it possible to determine internal flow fraction and consequently to develop a corrective factor for measurement. On the other hand, using 3-dimensional echocardiography makes it possible to estimate intraventricular volumes much more precisely than with the cross-sectional LV area.

Finally the use of this procedure should be verified in clinical studies.

11. References

[1] Suga H, Sagawa K, Shoukas AA. Load independence of the instantaneous pressure-volume ratio of the canine left ventricle and effects of epinephrine and heart rate on the ratio. Circ Res 1973;32:314-22.

[2] Gorcsan J, III, Morita S, Mandarino WA, et al. Two-dimensional echocardiographic automated border detection accurately reflects changes in left ventricular volume. J Am Soc Echocardiogr 1993;6:482-9.

[3] Deneault LG, Kancel MJ, Denault A, et al. A system for the on-line acquisition, visualization, and analysis of pressure-area loops. Comput Biomed Res 1994;27:61-7.

[4] Danielsen M, Ottesen JT. Describing the pumping heart as a pressure source. Journal of Theoretical Biology 2001;212:71-81.

[5] Ottesen JT, Danielsen M. Modeling ventricular contraction with heart rate changes. Journal of Theoretical Biology 2003;222:337-46.

[6] Paladino, J, Mulier, J, and Noordergraaf, A. Defining Ventricular Elastance. 1-11-0098.

[7] Strobeck JE, Sonnenblick EH. Myocardial and ventricular function. Part II: Intact heart. Herz 1981;6:275-87.

[8] Strobeck JE, Sonnenblick EH. Myocardial and ventricular function. Part I: Isolated muscle. Herz 1981;6:261-74.

[9] Frank O. Zur Dynamik des Herzmuskels. Z Biol 1895;32:370-447.

[10] Starling EH. The Linacre Lecture of the Law of the Heart. London: Longman, Greens and Co, Ltd, 1918.

[11] Seelen, P. J. A human circulatory analog computer. VIII Considerations leading to a preliminary analog of the left ventricle of the heart. 1961. Physics Lab, Univ. Utrecht. Ref Type: Internet Communication

[12] Beneken, J. E. W. A mathematical approach to cardio-vascular function. 1965. Univ. Utrecht. Ref Type: Thesis/Dissertation

[13] Liljestrand GLENG. The immediate effect of muscular work on the stroke and heart volume in man. Skand Arch Physiol 1938;80:265-82.

[14] Hill AV. The maximum work and mechanical efficiency of human muscles, and their most economical speed. J Physiol (London) 1922;56:19-41.

[15] Olufsen MS, Nadim A, Lipsitz LA. Dynamics of cerebral blood flow regulation explained using a lumped parameter model. Am J Physiol Regul Integr Comp Physiol 2002;282:R611-R622.

[16] Baan J, Jong TT, Kerkhof PL, et al. Continuous stroke volume and cardiac output from intra-ventricular dimensions obtained with impedance catheter. Cardiovasc Res 1981;15:328-34.

[17] Suga H, Sagawa K. Instantaneous pressure-volume relationships and their ratio in the excised, supported canine left ventricle. Circ Res 1974;35:117-26.

[18] Broscheit JA, Greim CA, Kessler M, Weidemann F, Roewer N: J Cardiothorac Vasc Anesth. 18(4): 415-22.

[19] Broscheit J, Greim CA, Weidemann F, Strotmann J, Steendijk P, Karle H, Roewer N: J Cardiothorac Vasc Anesth. 2006 Jun; 20(3): 340-346.

[20] Broscheit J, Weidemann F, Strotmann J, Steendijk P, Eberbach N, Karle H, Schuster F, Roewer N, Greim CA: J Cardiothorac Vasc Anesth Epub 2008 Jun 22.

[21] Weidemann F, Broscheit J, Eberbach N, Steendijk P, Voelker W, Greim C, Ertl G, Roewer N, Strotmann JM: Clin Sci (Lond). 2004 Feb; 106(2): 173-81.

[22] Broscheit JA, Weidemann F, Grein B, Lange M, Muellenbach R, Schuster F, Lindner C, Kunze E, Steendijk P, Roewer N, Greim CA: I Anesthesiology. 2009;18(1):1-16

[23] Broscheit JA, Rinck A, Anetseder M, Kessler M, Roewer N, Greim CA: J Cardiothorac Vasc Anesth. 2007 Feb;21(1):8-17

5

Electrical Heart Instability Evaluation in Conditions of Diastolic Heart Failure Suffered by Coronary Heart Disease Patients

E.P. Tatarchenko, N.V. Pozdnyakova, O.E. Morozova and E.A. Petrushin
Penza Extension Course Institute for Medical Practitioners
Russia

1. Introduction

In 1965 WHO experts singed out coronary heart disease (CHD) in a separate group. It was dictated by the growing epidemic incidence rate and high mortality from disease complications. Besides, it was urgent to take measures to treat the disease. However, the end of the XX century and the beginning of the XXI century have not brought any significant changes. The heart and vessel diseases complicated by atherosclerosis are still one of the main problems in most countries. The main reasons are high incidence of disease, stabile director disability and mortality among employable population. Each year, cardiovascular diseases cause 4.3 million deaths in Europe in general, and over 2 million in the EU, accounting for 48 and 42% of the total number of deaths respectively. Mortality from coronary heart disease among of men in the age of 65 is 3 times higher than among women. In older age mortality rate is equalized, and after 80 years of age it is 2 times higher among women.

In its essence, all the pathophysiological manifestations of coronary heart disease are caused by an imbalance between myocardial oxygen demand and oxygen delivery.

CHD may start abruptly with myocardial infarction (MI) or sudden cardiac death (SCD), but almost 50% of patients suffer immediately a chronic form of coronary heart disease. It is called exertional angina [2, 3]. In absolute figures it means approximately 30,000 – 40,000 patients with angina per 1 million population [4]. According to some reports men suffering angina live on average eight years less than those who do not have this pathology [5].

According to epidemiological studies, CHD patients suffer blood circulation blocking in most cases; it leads to approximately 90% sudden deaths. About half of patients with diagnosticated CHD die suddenly without a preceding pain syndrome.

Meanwhile, M.R.Cowie and others [2002] argue, the main risk factor for sudden death is left ventricular dysfunction. The prognosis of chronic heart failure (CHF) is still extremely serious, regardless of its etiology, but you should agree with J.N. Cohn and others [1999] who wrote that "...coronary disease may be an independent predictor of poor prognosis for patients suffering heart failure". Traditionally, CHF was considered to have connection with systolic dysfunction, however, in recent years the main subject of research of clinicians and physiologists is mechanisms of myocardium diastolic dysfunction (DD) development and its role in the onset of heart failure. Nowadays heart failure is considered as a syndrome which develops from various pathological heart changes, neuroendocrinal regulation disorders and represents a complex of circulatory reactions because of systolic or diastolic cardiac dysfunction.

About 50% of patients with chronic heart failure die within 5 years after the onset of clinical symptoms despite the use of combination therapy. According to the Framingham study, 75% of men with CHF and 62% of women die within 5 years after establishing diagnosis. Only half of patients with CHF die from heart failure which is refractory to therapy. The second half of patients with heart failure dies suddenly because of ventricular tachyarrhythmia. Oxymortia is the main death mechanism (in 30-80% of cases) among patients with CHF of II-III of functional class [8]. These facts allowed us to formulate an assumption that heart failure is the most the arrhythmogenic factor in cardiology and the most important sign of sudden death risk [9, 10].

Thus, the prediction and solution of sudden cardiac death (SCD) problem is only possible with the full study of the structural abnormalities and functional diseases which cause life-threatening arrhythmias acoording to modern model. Pathological changes of myocardium go with various dysfunctions of electrical heart activity. They are prognostically unfavorable in terms of the occurrence of fatally dangerous rhythm disturbances. The validity of the assumption is based on the fact that electrophysiological alternation of cells and cell membranes boosts the development of electrical heart instability (EHI) after the cases of transient coronary heart disease and myocardial infarction having developed in areas of myocardial dysfunction.

Though this problem is intensively investigated, the search of pathogenic mechanisms causing electrophysiological properties disorder and associated with pathological electrocardiographic and electrophysiological phenomena going with structural remodeling of myocardium in CHD is still important.

The research objective was to study the indicators characterizing electrical instability of myocardium suffered by CHD patients who have diastolic heart failure.

According to protocol adopted by local Ethical Committee a number of patients who had suffered myocardial infarction more than a year ago took part in the research. They had a stabile clinical course of coronary heart disease and clinical implications of chronic cardiac failure syndrome with left ventricle ejection fraction of 45% during the previous month. Each patient signed an agreement to take part in our research as a volunteer. We observed the group of 128 patients (36 women and 92 men). The average age of patients was 57.3±5.6 years.

The elimination criteria were coronary revascularization or cerebral stroke during the last 6 months, symptoms of VI class cardiac failure according to NYHA classification, clinically significant cardiac defects and lung diseases, dysfunctions of liver and nephros, atrial fibrillation.

Besides standard clinical research, we did the whole complex of work including electrocardiography in 12 derivations, echocardiography, Holter monitoring, registration of average signaling electrocardiography with identification of ventricular late potential, analysis of variability of cardiac rhythm, evaluation of ventricle repolarization-interval dispersion Q-T (QT_d), resolved interval Q-T (QT_C).

Electrical Heart Instability Evaluation in Conditions of Diastolic Heart Failure Suffered
by Coronary Heart Disease Patients

83

We evaluated left ventricular geometry and left atrium (end-diastolic size - EDD, size - ESD; end-systolic volume - EDV, end-systolic volume - ESV; left ventricular mass index – LVMI, relative thickness of the left ventricular wall; left atrium volume change index); left ventricular systolic function (ejection fraction - EF, %; stroke index – SI, ml/m²; systolic shortening`s fraction of the front-back size aortic ventricle - ΔS,%); myocardium regional contractility (diacrisis of zone with regional contractility dysfunction). We used ultrasound cordis investigation with Doppler spectral echocardiography mode and color Doppler mapping.

Analyzing left ventricular diastolic function we studied indeces of transmitral diastolic flow in incipient and delayed diastole (E, A, m/s), their ratio (E/A), time of flow delay(DT, ms) and flow acceleration during the phase of rapid inflow(AT, ms), is ovolumic relaxation time (IVRT, ms) and duration of diastole (ET, ms) - Figure 1.

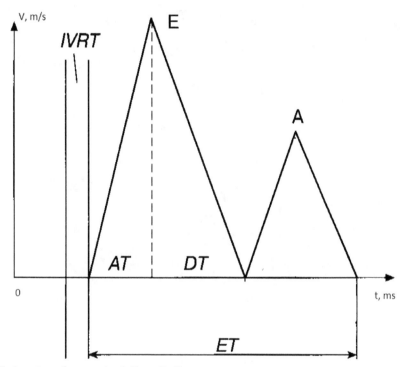

Fig. 1. Estimation of trancmitral diastolic flow

We also evaluated blood flow at the mouth of the pulmonary veins (D, cm / s; Ar, cm / s; Adur / Ar) – Figure 2.

We used tissue Doppler sonography to detect signs of inflow disorder, loss of elasticity, the increase of the left ventricular rigidity. We defined the maximum speed of mitral annulus: peak systolic speed - S '(cm / s) peak speed of incipient diastolic relaxation - E' (cm / s) peak speed in atrial systole phase - A '(cm / s), the ratio of maximum speed of incipient LV inflow (E) to the maximum speed of the fibrous ring kinesis in incipient diastole (E') - Figure 3.

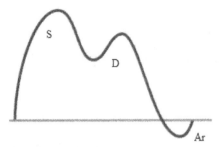

Fig. 2. Estimation of bloodstream at the mouth of the pulmonary veins

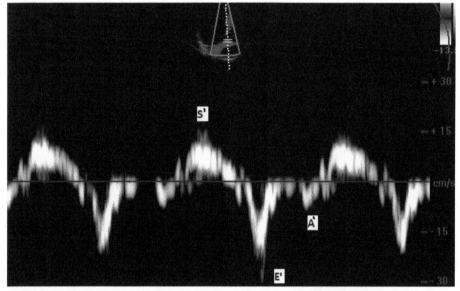

S' (cm/s) – peak diastolic speed; E' (cm/s) – peak speed of incipient diastolic relaxation; A' (cm/s) – peak speed in atrial systole phase.

Fig. 3. Fibrous ring`s movement of the mitral valve in pulse-wave mode histic doppler

Using Holter monitoring ECG we took into account the nature of rhythm disturbance and asequence, we estimated the quantity of pain assessed and painless ischemic episodes, the daily duration of ischemia, the maximum depth of segment ST depression.

Time-line analysis of ventricular late potential was performed by method of M. Simson [1981]. We calculated numerical quantitative values of three indicators: the duration of the filtered complex QRS (HF QRS-Dauer), the rms amplitude of the last 40 ms of the complex QRS (RMS 40), the duration of the low amplitude signals at the end of the filtered complex QRS (LAH Fd). We took HF QRS-Dauer which is more than 114 ms, RMS 40 which is less than 25 mV, LAH Fd which is more than 38 ms as pathological parameters of the signal averaged ECG - Figure 4.

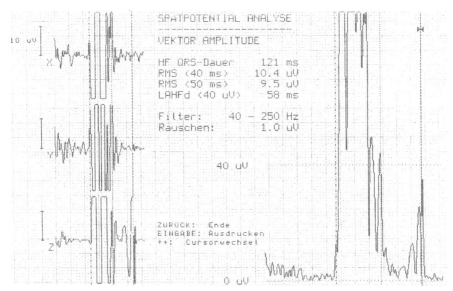

Fig. 4. Analysis of the signal-averaged ECG with elimination late potentials of the ventricles

Performing heart rate variability analysis we evaluated rMSSD (mean square difference between the duration of contiguous sinus intervals RR, BB 50 (proportion of contiguous sinus intervals RR which differ more than 50ms,%), SDNN (standard derivation of average duration of sinus intervals RR, ms).

Performing spectral analysis of heart rate variability analysis we estimated frequency ranges: high frequency (HF), low frequency (LF), the ratio of sympathetic and parasympathetic influences on heart rate variability (LF/HF).

We examined the following heart rate turbulence indicants:

- turbulence onset (TO,%). We estimated the value-of sinus rhythm acceleration after ventricular arrhythmia;
- turbulence slope (TS, ms / RR). We studied the intensity of the sinus rhythm deceleration, following its quickening.

In assessing ventricular repolarization we calculated corrected interval Q-T (QTs) using Bazeta. The dispersion of the interval Q-T (QTd) was defined as the difference between the maximal and minimal value of Q-T interval in different leads of standard ECG.

T-test of Student, entry criteria applied by static data handing. Gotten results have been presented in the form of an average arithmetical significance ± is standart devition. Differences considered reliable at $p < 0,05$.

In case of CHD left ventricle diastole indices and diastole functions undergo complex changes which are connected with both worsening of diastolic disorders and the development of hemodynamic adaptive responses acting through an increase in pressure in the left atrium and/or left ventricular end diastolic pressure and leading to the formation of various types of diastolic dysfunction.

We divided our patients into 3 groups according to the type of diastolic dysfunction of left ventricle: the first group (n=36) included patients with abnormal relaxation of left ventricle, the second group (n=28) consisted of patients with pseudonormal type of diastolic dysfunction and the third group (n=22) was formed from the patients who suffered restrictive type of diastolic dysfunction of left ventricle.

The average duration of disease was 6.9 ± 3.9 years (3 to 12 years). Medical history and electrocardiographic criteria indicated macrofocal myocardial infarction (with Q tooth) suffered by 68 patients (53.1%).9 out of 68 patients had a chronic aneurysm of the anterior wall according to electrocardiographic and echocardiographic features. Fine-focal MI (without Q tooth) is marked in 60 cases according to medical documentation (hospital records, discharge summary). 82 patients (64%) had coronary heart disease accompanied by arterial hypertension (AH). 92 patients (72%) had burdened familial history. Lipid exchange violations were indicated in 112 cases (87.5%).

Figure 1 shows the gradation of patients with different variants of the left ventricle diastolic dysfunction according to functional classes of chronic heart failure (CHF). 42 patients had signs of I FC CHF, 51 patients had II FC and 35 patients had III FC.

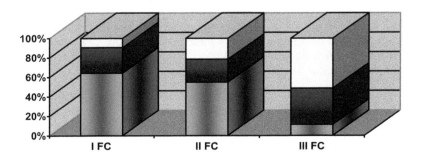

◩ diastolic dysfunction of abnormal relaxation type   ◼ pseudonormal type of diasto
◻ restrictive type of diastolic dysfunction

Fig. 5. The gradation of patients suffering coronary heart disease with left ventricle diastolic dysfunction according to functional classes of chronic heart failure (CHF).

In cases of heart failure clinical manifestations we have received the relation of r = 0,620 (p <0.01) of the frequency of CHF FC to the type of diastolic dysfunction. When FC increases the disturbances of LV DF become more pronounced: restrictive type of LV DD was detected in III FC (51% observations); in I FC it was observed on 11.4%; patients had the type of abnormal relaxation in 9.5% and 64.3% respectively, pseudonormal type was detected in 21.6% and 55% of cases.

The analysis of the structural and geometric parameters of left heart chambers (Table 1) showed that group III had an increase of the dilation of the cavities of the left ventricle and left atrium, increased left ventricle myocardial mass, reduction in contractile function (ejection fraction of III group was more than 45% but less than 50%, in group I it was 50%) in comparison with group I.

Indicators	I group	II group	III group
Number of patients, n	59	36	33
E, m/s	0.65±0.06*	0.81±0.03	1.07±0.05**
A, m/s	0.93±0.09*	0.65±0.02	0.36±0.03*
E/A,	0.82±0.05*	1.25±0.02	3.15±0.08**
AT, ms	99.47±2.1	94.1±3.2	97.3±3.3
DT, ms	267.6±11.4*	169.6±7.9	143.5±3.2**
IVRT, ms	116.8±7.4*	88.3±2.3	58.9±4.8**
Ar, cm/s	24.1±2.2°	36.6±1.3	55.3±1.6
SI, ml/m²	40.3±2.8	41.2±1.4	41.7±2.6
EDVI, ml/m²	82.1±5.3*	85.8±4.58	100.8±6.7
ESVI, ml/m²	37.85±2.1*	39.2±1.1	41.61±2.5
LVEF, %	55.93±2.7*	53.1±2.17	49.6±2.06
ESVILA, ml/m²	39.5±2.3*	44.37±3.2	50.43±3.61
ICVLA,%	37.65±1.5 *	34.1±2.1	24.9±2.7
LVMI, g/m²	126.35±9.7*	132.1±6.3	148.2±11.1
left ventricular RT, cm	0.44±0.06*	0.45±0.05	0.50±0.02

SI – stroke index, EDVI - end-diastolic volume index, ESVI - end systolic volume index, LVEF - left ventricular ejection fraction, ESVILA - end systolic volume index of left atrium, the ICVLA - an indicator of changes in the volume of the left atrium, LVMI - left ventricular mass index, left ventricular RT is the relative thickness of the left ventricular wall, *-p <0.05 - reliability of differences between patients with DD of abnormal relaxation type and patients with pseudonormal type of DD, ** p <0.05 - reliability of differences between the group of patients with restrictive type of DD and the groups with pseudonormal type of DD and abnormal relaxation, ° - p <0.05 - reliability of the indicator difference between group with DD of abnormal relaxation type and groups with DD of pseudonormal and restrictive type.

Table 1. Echocardiographic indicators of patients with coronary heart disease

We believe that one of the determinants of heart failure is diastolic dysfunction of the heart, which can be viewed both as the initial stage and as a pathophysiological link in the "vicious circle" of circulatory inefficiency, which affects negatively on the prognosis of patients with coronary heart disease [11].

The violation of left ventricular diastolic properties is essential, along with other structural and functional changes (dilation and hypertrophy), which form the concept of "remodeling". Patients had eccentric hypertrophy (43.75% of cases) and concentric hypertrophy of LV (37.5% of cases) as predominant types of LV remodeling after MI.

We established the correlation between the severity of LV DD and exponent change in the volume of the left atrium - r = -0.43 (p = 0.032), with left ventricular ejection fraction - r = -0.48 (p <0.04), with an index of end diastolic volume - r = 0,51 (p = 0.02), with left ventricular mass index - r = 0.45 (p = 0.034).

We associate the appearance and progression of LV DD with violation of diastolic relaxation on the back of acute or long-lasting ischemia with increased stiffness of the myocardium, including the location of postinfarction scar. We spotted the following law: a degree of LV DF disorder was growing in patients having macrofocal myocardial infarction versus patients having fine-focal myocardial infarction, respectively, it was 30.5% with abnormal relaxation type and 69.5% (p = 0.047), 58.3% and 41.7% (p = 0.05) with pseudonormal, 87.9% and 12.1% (p = 0.0476) with restrictive type. We believe that patients with previous Q-infarction had long-lasting deterioration of LV function during myocardial hibernating, which is characterized by a chronic reduction in cardiomyocyte contractility, while their viability is maintained. In these conditions viable myocardium which is far from infarction zona undergoes diastolic myocardial stress.

We detected the dependence of manifestation degree of diastolic dysfunction with an index of contractility WMSI - r = 0.91 (p = 0.01) among patients with a history of MI. We pointed the positive correlation of restrictive type of LV DD with Q- myocardial infarction r = 0.638 (p <0.001). In group III (restrictive type) Q-infarction occurred in 87.9% of cases, which is significantly lower in comparison with group I – 30.5%, p <0.01.

In conditions of limited blood flow the possibility of injury and death of cardiomyocytes because of their necrotization and apoptosis [12] is the main unfavorable result of myocardial hypoxia in case of coronary heart disease. However, death of cardiomyocytes is accompanied by compensatory hypertrophy of survived myocardial cell and the development of connective tissue [13]. There is an opinion that left ventricle hypertrophy may lead to myocardial dysfunction. It is an individual risk factor for high cardiovascular case rate, including ischemia myocardial infarction, heart failure, ventricular arrhythmias and sudden death.

We tend to assume that the process of cardiac remodeling affects all myocardium components. Changes occur at the level of cardiac myocytes and in the extracellular matrix. Typically, ischemic myocardial injuries develop leading to the coagulation and apoptosis. In this case, as approved by the J.Soto, G.Beller [2001], responsive genes are activated immediately, especially c-fos, and the program of "programmed death", apoptosis, starts to run. In the peripheral areas ischemic injury usually results in colliquative necrosis with cell edema and myocytolysis. It is especially true for reperfusion injury. The formation of connective tissue (fibrosis) may have redundant diffuse or interstitial nature in addition to substitution (focal), with interstitial spread perivascular.

Different biomechanical properties of myocardium in chronic ischemic zone and so-called intact myocardium generate special effects according to the type of stress concentration on their border. The type of stress concentration is connected with further progression of degenerative and sclerotic changes, significant changes in the shape and size of remodeled heart chambers. Further LV remodeling with the expansion of the cavity in postinfarction period is caused by involving of myocardium in the "transition zone" in the process of remodeling. The data obtained from pathophysiological studies suggest that patients suffering coronary heart disease have clinical picture determined by not only the heterogeneity of causes, but also the diversity of adaptive and disadaptive changes in metabolism and contractile condition of cardiomyocytes [16]. The most significant adaptive myocardium reactions in response to myocardial ischemia include the "new ischemic syndromes": hibernate, stupor.

The defining condition for the occurrence of lethal arrhythmias is considered to be structural disease of heart, which becomes electrically unstable under the influence of various functional factors. Ischemia and necrosis, hypertrophy and dilatation of the ventricles, the inflammation and swelling of the myocardial tissue can act as the structural changes that determine the development of ventricular tachycardia. According to the results of many studies [17, 18, 19] these changes constitute anatomical substrate for appearance of malignant arrhythmias with the participation of the various triggering and modulating factors.

Ventricular late potential with a stable disease course was recorded among 35 patients (27.3%) with a history of MI (Table 2). We believe that structural cardiomyocyte changes, programmed apoptosis and secondary hypertrophy, increased diastolic stiffness and active myocardium relaxation violation, reactive changes of connective tissue skeleton of the myocardium, decrease in diastolic filling and remodeling with segmental structure violation, i.e. all these processes, lead to the formation of electrical myocardium heterogeneity and cause greater frequency of recording of late potentials among CHD patients in conditions of progression of LV DD: with abnormal relaxation (18.6%), with pseudonormal type (27.8%), and restrictive type of LV DD (42.4%, p <0.05).

Indicator	Variations of diastolic dysfunction		
	Type I	Type II	Type III
The number of patients, n	59	36	33
The number of patients with ventricle late potential, n	11	10	14
The number of patients with ventricular arrhythmia, n	50	35	33
analysis of ventricular extrasystole			
I gradation, n/%	29/49.1%	10/27.8%	2/6.1%
IIgradation, n/%	7/11.9%	7/19.4%	5/15.1%
IIIgradation, n/%	10/16.9%	13/36.1%	12/36.4%
IV-V gradations, n/%	4/6.8%	5/13.9%	14/42.4%
analysis of Q-T interval			
RRNN, ms	810 ± 64	798 ± 98	753 ± 132
QT$_c$, ms	405.5 ± 5.2*	422.3 ± 2.6**	450.2 ± 5.4
QT$_d$, ms	39.7 ± 2.7*	49.6 ± 3.3**	64.2 ± 3.1

I type- LV DD of abnormal relaxation type, II type - LV DD of pseudonormal type; III type - LV DD of restrictive type, VLP ventricular late potential, VA- ventricular arrhythmia, RRNN - the duration of sinus RR intervals; n /% - the absolute number of patients with given symptom/percentage of the number of patients of this group.

Table 2. The comparative analysis of ventricular arrhythmias, cardiac late potentials, QT intervals among patients with coronary heart disease

Ventricular arrhythmias are considered to be one of the factors determining the poor prognosis and high mortality among CHD patients. Ventricular arrhythmias may be the cause of death among patients with heart failure symptoms even in conditions of adequate control of decompensation symptoms.

Cardiac arrhythmias were detected among 99.2% of patients (Table 2), while supraventricular arrhythmias (SA) were detected among 7% of patients, ventricular arrhythmias were detected among 56.2% of patients, a combination of ventricular arrhythmias (VA) with various forms of supraventricular arrhythmias (SA) were indicated among 36% of patients. Complex forms of VA (ventricular extrasystole of grades IV-V) were found in 23 cases (18%). Polymorphic ventricular extrasystole was detected among 35 CHD patients with left ventricular diastolic dysfunction (27.3%). In 41 cases (32%) the revealed ventricular extrasystole was assigned to I gradation when the frequency of episodes did not exceed 220 per day.

Having analyzed ventricular arrhythmias we noted the following law: early, paired, volley ventricular extrasystoles were detected among patients with slow fragmented activity more frequently in comparison with patients without ventricular late potential, respectively, 19 (54.3%) and 4 (4.3%) with $\chi2 = 7.4$, p <0.001.

Ventricular late potential and ventricular arrhythmias were recorded more often with an increase in the degree of diastolic dysfunction and end-diastolic volume of left ventricle. When DD had a restrictive type, ventricular extrasystole was found in 100% of cases and ventricular extrasystole of IV-V grades was detected among 14 patients (42.4%), 13 of them had a diagnosed slow fragmented activity at the end of the ventricular complex. In group I (with abnormal left ventricular relaxation) ventricular extrasystole was observed among 84.7% of patients and complex forms of ventricular extrasystole were detected among 4 patients with abnormal rates of Holter ECG (6.8%).

The most common mechanism for tachyarrhythmias of high grades is the mechanism of re-entry momentum. It means the presence of unilateral and delayed passage of the depolarization wave front because of the violation of inter-cell contacts in parallel-oriented fibers [20], proliferation heterogeneity and fragmentation of the depolarization wavefront, which is a marked by ventricular late potential. That's what we explain the significant prevalence of complex forms of ventricular extrasystole among patients with slow fragmented ventricular activity (54.3%).

To study the effect of reversible ischemia on myocardial electrophysiological properties we analyzed daily myocardial ischemia and indicators of Holter ECG among patients with coronary heart disease having left ventricular DD. Correlation analysis revealed the dependence of the daily duration of ischemia on the duration of filtered set of HF QRS Dauer (r = 0.53, p = 0.01), with duration of low-amplitude signals at the end of filter-centered complex QRS LAH Fd (r = 0.49 p = 0.03), duration of painless myocardial ischemia with HF QRS Dauer (r = 0.57, p = 0.01). A positive correlation was obtained by estimating the depth of segment depression in HF QRS-Dauer (r = 0.45, p = 0.03), with LAH Fd (r = 0.41, p = 0.05); number of painless ischemic episodes per day with HF QRS-Dauer (r = 0.51, p = 0.04).

The results confirm that the presence of slow fragmented activity focus, marked by ventricular late potential is connected with heterogeneous areas of myocardium in CHD patients: profound disturbances in the processes of relaxation and recovery of cardiomyocytes occur in both acute and chronic ischemia because of degenerative changes and apoptosis. But it should be noted that studying the complex mechanisms of late potentials formation and the functions and metabolism of cardiac muscle, we traditionally pay much attention to cardiomyocytes. However, we tend to assume that extracellular matrix plays a insignificant role in the genesis of fragmented ventricular activity. Fibrosis is an essential component of cardiac muscle remodeling; the development of reparative (replacement) fibrosis may not only violate cardiomyocytes supply but also impede the electrical contact between them [21] in case of ischemia and myocardial necrosis.

The results of our studies have shown that myocardial dysfunction in ischemic area leads to the inhomogeneity of repolarization processes in conditions of limited coronary blood flow. However, the increase of QT dispersion in patients with coronary heart disease is associated with the duration of daily myocardial ischemia (DMI). We received a positive relationship of DMI with QT_d (r = 0.485, p = 0.05). When the DMI was more than 60 minutes the duration of QTc and QT_d interval was 449.2±4.1 ms and 67.2±2.7ms, p <0.05,when the DMI was 30 to 60 min analogous figures corresponded to the values of 412.5±3,2ms and 46.8± 2,4 ms.

While studying QTd we observed higher values in patients with ventricular arrhythmia of III-V grades (67.5±4.2 ms) in comparison with patients without ventricular arrhythmia (44.3±2.5ms), p <0,05. The analysis revealed a dependence of the variance of QT interval with gradation of ventricular extrasystole (r = 0.6432, p <0.01), with exponents of Holter ECG: LAH Fd (r = 0.4831, p <0.05) HF QRS-Dauer (r = 0.5744, p <0.05).

The proportion of patients with restrictive type of LV DD with QTc interval which was over 440 ms (69%), and QTd which was more than 50 ms (72%) was significantly higher in comparison with those values in group II, it was 30.6% and 33% (p<0.05) respectively, and in Group I it was 19% and 17% (p<0.03) respectively.

The performance analysis of electrical and structural remodeling among patients havingcoronary heart disease with different variants of left ventricular DD allowed us to establish a clear pattern (Figure 6): ventricular late potential and ventricular arrhythmias of higher grades were detected more often with increasing degree of diastolic function disturbance. Inhomogeneity of repolarization processes was heightened with an increase in QT interval dispersion. In our view, the resulting dependence reflects inhomogeneity of repolarization processes and depolarization of the ventricles in chronic ischemia, the conditions for malignant arrhythmias in CHD patients having left ventricular DD were created. We assume that the electrical stability of myocardium and its global-sustaining capacity are integral characteristics that determine the functioning of the heart as a self-regulating system. The violation of bioelectrical activity of the myocardium inevitably leads to its mechanical failure.

The discussion of the pathogenesis of coronary heart disease was always connected with neurogenic component. The theory of "punctuated antagonism" of the interaction of two divisions of the autonomic nervous system (ANS) and their impact on the regulation of the pacemaker in the sinus node (SN) is complicated by the activity of all the structures of the peripheral segmental heart ANS. In conditions of limited coronary blood flow morpho-functional component is considered to be slowly-varied, and pathologically altered regulation of heart rate variability is one of the earliest and most obligate manifestations of ischemic process [22, 23]. Sympathetic distress is a critical drop in power of neurohumoral regulation with a shift in the sympathovagal balances to the sympathetic component. It is regarded as a predictor of sudden death which is independent from left ventricular ejection fraction [22].

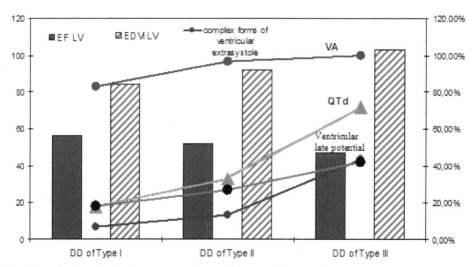

DD of Type I - diastolic dysfunction according to the type of abnormal relaxation, DD of Type II-diastolic dysfunction of pseudonormal type, DD of Type III - diastolic dysfunction of restrictive type; EDVI LV - end-diastolic volume index of left ventricle, EF LV - ejection fraction left ventricular, QTd - the dispersion of Q-T interval.

Fig. 6. The performance analysis of structural and geometrical and eletrical remodeling in CHD patients with left ventricle diastolic dysfunction.

Assessing the neurohumoral regulation of heart rate, we conducted the analysis of quantitative indicators of HRV and HRT (Table 3).

HRV indices in the group with impaired relaxation did not differ significantly from those in the group with pseudonormal type, once-reliable differences were obtained in comparison with III group of diastolic heart failure.

Rates BB50, SDNN index, rMSSD are drastically reduced in patients of group III. These values indicate a disorder of vagal protective effect on the value of "threshold of heart fibrillation". Disorders of neurohumoral regulation were diagnosed in conditions of the restrictive version of the DD LV, they pointed the increased sympathetic activity (SDNN – 24.7±3,2ms, LF/HF – 5.46±0,61 conventional units, BB50 - 0%).

During our study we pointed out the following pattern: autonomic imbalance with increased sympathetic activity grew with an increase in the degree of LV DD. The excess of

Electrical Heart Instability Evaluation in Conditions of Diastolic Heart Failure Suffered
by Coronary Heart Disease Patients

93

the balance of ANS of sympathetic type LF / HF was observed in 39% of patients in group I who had abnormal left ventricular relaxation, it was detected in 58.3% of patients in group II with pseudonormal type of DD LV and it was indicated in 94% cases in group III with restrictive type, p <0.05.

And, if the HRV is a proven non-invasive method of quantitative analysis of the functioning of ANS in patients with coronary heart disease with preserved sinus rhythm, HRT is a fairly new noninvasive method of estimation the modulating autonomic influences on the sinus node in patients with ventricular arrhythmias, which resulted from the progressive fading of the carotid baroreflex [24]. Schematically, the formation of HRT can be represented by the following sequence: compensatory pause occurs after ventricular extrasystole, and, as a result, heart rate and blood pressure increase are caused by baroreflex, then blood pressure increase leads to the subsequent decrease in heart rate through baroreflex.

Indicators	Group I	Group II	Group III
The number of patients, n	59	36	33
RRNN, ms	810±64	798 ± 98	753 ± 132
analysis of heart rate variability			
SDNN, ms	41.4± 2.7	36.6± 2.3	24.7± 3.2*
SDNN index, ms	22.6 ±1.9	19.3 ±1.3	8.7±1.6*
rMSSD, ms	23.1±2.1	21.1±1.4	16 ±1.3*
BB50, beats per minute	10.3±3.2	8.8±1.4	3.4±1.2*
LF/HF, conv.	2.93±0.54	3.51±0.68	5.16 ±0.61*
analysis of heart rate turbulence			
TO more 0% , n/ %	10/17	9/25	17/51.5
TS less 2,5мс/RR, n/ %	9/15.2	9/25	16/48.5

RRNN - the average duration of sinus RR intervals between contractions, SDNN-standard deviation from the mean duration of RR intervals between sinus contractions, BB50 - the number of adjacent sinus RR intervals, which differ by more than 50 ms, SDNN index-average standard deviations, rMSSD - square root of the sum of squared differences of successive sinus RR intervals, LF/HF - index of the balance of sympathetic and parasympathetic nervous systems; TO is more than 0%; TS is less than 2.5 ms / RR * - p <0, 05 – the difference is reliable when indicators of group III are compared with indicators of I and II groups.

Table 3. Quantitative indices of HRV in patients with coronary heart disease

HRT indicators reflect early acceleration of sinus rhythm (TO) and the subsequent decrease in heart rate (TS) after ventricular arrhythmia. Studies in recent years characterized HRT as effective method of predicting the outcomes of patients with coronary pathology, which is comparable with HRV, and in some cases it is superior to HRV in its diagnostic capabilities [25, 26].

During our study we reported the value of TO> 0% in 36 patients (28%) from the group of 128 patients with previous MI history, we detected TS <2.5 ms / RR in 34 cases (26.6%), and we observed the combination of pathological values of TO and TS in 19 cases (14.8%). The frequency of registration TO> 0% and TS <2.5 ms / RR significantly dominated in the group with restrictive type of LV DD in comparison with group I (DD type of abnormal relaxation) and group II (DD of pseudonormal type), p <0.05.

We have established a connection of HRT violation with left atrium volume change indicator- r = -0.43 (p = 0.032), with left ventricular ejection fraction- r = -0.49 (p =0.03), with end-diastolic volume index - r = 0.51 (p = 0.02), with left ventricular mass index - r = 0.45 (p = 0.04). We marked the correlation of TS with HRV indicators: SDNN (r = 0.41, p = 0.02) and LH/HF (r = 0.332, p = 0.02). The absolute values of TO significantly correlated with QTd (r = 0.349, p = 0.04).

Pathophysiologic ground for coronary heart disease is a discrepancy between myocardial oxygen demand and opportunities in meeting the needs in oxygen because of a limitation of acute or chronic coronary blood flow. Admittedly, the provision of myocardial blood through the coronary arteries occurs in the phase of diastole. That is why we suggest to consider diastolic dysfunction not only as an initial stage, but also as a pathological link in the "vicious circle" of the development of cardiac events in CHD patients.

Rates of diastole and its function undergo complex changes caused by the violation of diastolic relaxation in the background of acute or chronic ischemia, with increased stiffness of the myocardium at the site of postinfarction scar during the coronary heart disease. Necrosis of cardiomyocytes and activation of the cascade of biochemical reactions which occur in the postinfarction period, cause a significant change in mechanical properties of tissues. However, we should take into account different biomechanical properties of myocardium in the areas of chronic ischemia and so-called intact (healthy) myocardium. The specific effects are generated on their borders according to the type of stress concentration. They cause the further progression of degenerative and sclerotic changes, the formation of connective tissue in conditions of limited blood flow. In conditions of chronic ischemia, the changes occur not only in cardiomyocytes but also in cells of connective tissue skeleton. Increased rigidity of myocardium, change in the myocardium viscoelastic properties are the consequences of disorganization and reorganization of connective tissue skeleton of ischemic nature. Progressive hypertrophy and dilation of the heart are accompanied by a further violation of the diastolic left ventricular function, then it is accompanied by systolic dysfunction, they cause an increase in myocardial oxygen demand and a change in subendocardial blood flow, impaired myocardial bioenergetics.

The evaluation of the changes of myocardium electrophysiological properties seems for us to be an important aspect in the search for new diagnostic tests of severity of ischemic myocardial damage in patients with coronary heart disease. The validity of these approaches is based on the notion that electrophysiological alternation of cells and their membranes is associated with remodeling after an episode of ischemia or myocardial infarction and is involved in genesis of arrhythmia That is why we examined the relationship of electrical and structural myocardium remodeling with left ventricular diastolic function in CHD patients who had myocardial infarction history.

The analysis of ventricular late potentials and dispersion of QT interval allows to assess arrhythmogenic substrate in patients having CHD with left ventricular diastolic dysfunction. Persistent deterioration of left ventricular diastolic function during myocardium hibernating among CHD patients increases the manifestation of inhomogeneity of depolarization and repolarization processes.

The increase of the sympathetic influence has an effect on myocardium active relaxation and diastolic phase structure during the subsequent abuse of metabolic pathways accompanied by destabilization of connective tissue skeleton and secondary changes of contractile myocardium. Neurohumoral regulation violations caused by diastolic dysfunction in CHD patients are the same as when they are generated by heart failure. They are evident in increase of sympathetic activity, reduced parasympathetic and pressosensitive activity.

Even single ventricular extrasystole can be a trigger factor of fatally dangerous arrhythmias in conditions of chronic myocardial ischemia with arrhythmogenic substrate, which is the marked by ventricular late potential and QTd, when autonomic nervous system is activated according to the sympathetic type.

Complex analysis of parameters reflecting the functional conditions of myocardium and the interrelation of electrical and structure-geometrical myocardium remodeling is necessary to improve the diagnostics and the prognostication of risk degree among CHD patients in conditions of increasing of left ventricle diastolic dysfunction, given the multifactorial genesis of the problem of myocardial electrical instability

The use of integrated risk markers may contribute to the development of an integrated approach to risk stratification of SCD and arrhythmic complications prevention in CHD patients.

2. Abbreviations

ANS - autonomic nervous system

CHD - coronary heart disease

CHF - chronic heart failure

DD - diastolic dysfunction

DF - diastolic function

EDD - end-diastolic size

EDV - end-diastolic volume

ESD - end- systolic size

EHI - electrical heart instability

ESV - end- systolic volume

EF - ejection fraction

HRT - heart rate turbulence

HRV - heart rate variability

IVRT – isovolumic relaxation time

LV - left ventricle

LVMI - left ventricular mass index

MI - myocardial infarction

SA - supraventricular arrhythmias

SCD - sudden cardiac death

SI – stroke index

ΔS - systolic shortening's fraction of the front-back size aortic ventricle

VA - ventricular arrhythmia

VLP - ventricular late potential

3. References

[1] Allender S., Scarborough P., Peto V., Rayner M., Leal J., Luengo-Fernandez R., Gray A. . European cardiovascular disease statistics 2008 // Eur. Heart Network. -2008.- Vol. 4. – P. 76–78.

[2] Kannel W.B., Feinleib M. Natural history of angina pectoris in the Framingham study. Prognosis and survival // American Journal of Cardiology. – 1972.- Vol. 29.- P. 154-163.

[3] Pepine C.J., Abrams J., Marks R.G. et al. Characteristics of a contemporary population with angina pectoris: TIDES Investigators // Am. J. Cardiol. – 1994.- Vol. 74.- P. 226-231.

[4] Williams S.V., Fihn S.D., Gibbons R.J. Guidelines for the management of patients with chronic stable angina: diagnosis and risk stratification// Ann. Intern. Med. – 2001.- Vol. 135.- P. 530-547.

[5] Oganov R.G., Maslennikova. G.Y. Demographic situation and cardiovascular diseases in Russia: ways to solve problems// Cardiovascular therapies and prevention. .- 2007.- №6. – P.7-14.

[6] Cowie M.R., Fox K.F., Wood D.A. et al. Hospitalization of patients with heart failure: a population–based study. //Eur Heart J. - 2002.- Vol. 23.- P. 877–85.

[7] Cohn, J.N., Johnson G. Veterans Administration Cooperative Study Group. Heart failure with normal ejection fraction: V-HEFT Study // Circulation. - 1990.- Vol. 81.- P. 48-53.

[8] O'Callaghan P.A., Camm A.J. Treatment of arrhythmias in heart failure // Europ. J. Heart Failure.- 1999.- Vol.1 (2).- P. 133-137.

Electrical Heart Instability Evaluation in Conditions of Diastolic Heart Failure Suffered
by Coronary Heart Disease Patients

97

[9] Mareev V.Y. Heart failure and ventricular arrhythmias: the problem of treatment.//
Cardiology.-1996.- № 12.- P.4–12.

[10] Cowie M.R., Mosterd A., Wood D.A. et al. The epidemiology of heart failure // Eur
Heart J. – 1997. - Vol. 18.- P. 208-255.

[11] Devereux R.B. Left ventricular diastolic dysfunction: early diastolic relaxation and late
diastolic compliance. J. Am. Coll. Cardiol 1989; 13: 337-339.

[12] Kapelko V.E. The evolution of concepts and metabolic basis of ischemic myocardial
dysfunction.// Cardiology. - 2005. - № 9. – P. 55–61.

[13] Wainwright C.L. Matrix metalloproteinases? Oxidative stress and the acute response to
acute myocardial ischemia-reperfusion // Curr Opin Pharmacol. - 2004.- Vol. 4.-
P. 132 – 138.

[14] Molkentin J.D., Lu J-R, Antos C.L. et al. A calcineurin-dependent transcriptional
pathway for cardiac hypertrophy // Cell.- 1998. – Vol. 93.- P. 215 - 228.

[15] Soto J., Beller G. Clinical Benefit of Noninvasive Viability Studies of Patients with
Severe Ischemic Left Ventricular Dysfunction // Clin. Cardiol. – 2001. - Vol. 24. - P.
428-434.

[16] Opie L.H. Newly identified ischemic syndromes and myocardial endogenous
cytoprotection and their role in clinical cardiology in the past and future. //
Medicography. - 1999. - № 21(2). - P. 65–73.

[17] Hohnloser S.H., Franck P., Klingenheben T. et al. Open infarct artery, late potentials,
and other prognostic factors in patients after acute myocardial infarction in the
thrombolytic era: a prospective trial // Circulation. – 1994.- Vol, 90.- P. 1747-1756.

[18] Goldstein S., Brooks M. M., Ledingham R. et al. Association between ease of
suppression of ventricular arrhythmia and survival// Circulation. – 1995.- Vol. 91.-
P. 7979 – 7983.

[19] Petersen S., Peto V., Rayner M. et al. European cardiovascular disease statistics // Eur.
Heart J. – 2005. - Vol. 21. - P. 1261-1272.

[20] Kramer J.B., Saffitz J.E., Witkowsky F.V., Corr P.B. Intramural reentry as a mechanism
of ventriculartachycardia during evolving canine myocardial infarction.// Circ.
Res.- 1985 - Vol. 56 - P. 736-754.

[21] Tatarchenko E.P., Pozdnyakova N.V., Morozova O.E. Late potentials of the heart:
clinical and electrophysiological evaluation. Penza: Elma.- 2000. – P. 144 .

[22] Maisch B. Ventricular remodeling // Cardiology.- 1996.- Vol. 8(7).- P. 2-10.

[23] Bigger J., Fleiss J.L., Steiman R.C. Correlation among time and freguency domain
measures of heart period variability two week after acute myocardial infarction.
Am. J. Cardiol 1992; 69: 891 - 898.

[24] Tatarchenko E.P., Pozdnyakova N.V., Morozova O.E., Shevyryov V.A. Prognosis of
patients with coronary heart disease (clinical and instrumental aspects). Penza:
Elma.- 2002. – P. 206.

[25] Schmidt G., Malik M., Barthel P. et al. Heart-rate turbulence after ventricular premature
beats as a predictor of mortality after acute myocardial infarction // Lancet.- 1999.-
Vol.353.- P.1390-1396.

[26] Ghuran A., Reid F., La Rovere M.T. et al. Heart rate turbulence-based predictors of fatal and nonfatal cardiac arrest (The Autonomic Tone and Reflexes After Myocardial Infarction substudy) // Am. J. Cardiol.- 2002.- Vol.89.- P.184-190

[27] Bauer A., Barthel P., Schneider R., Schmidt G. Dynamics of heart rate turbulence // Circulation.- 2001.- Vol.104, Supplement II-339.- P.1622.

Part 3

Pharmacotherapy of Ischemic Heart Disease

6

Thrombolysis in Myocardial Infarction

Ajay Suri[1], Sophia Tincey[2],
Syed Ahsan[1] and Pascal Meier[1]
[1]The Heart Hospital, University College Hospital, London
[2]North Middlesex Hospital, London
UK

1. Introduction

Worldwide around 7 million people suffer myocardial infarctions per year according to White et al. (2008). Around one third of these patients having acute myocardial infarction die within the first hour of having symptoms usually due to fatal arrhythmia. Characteristic ST segment elevation in the 12 lead electrocardiogram (ECG) accompanied by clinical symptoms of chest pain provide the most rapid way to diagnose those patients who should receive thrombolysis to help dissolve thrombus and restore blood flow. In fact, since the early 1980s, thombolysis has been the cornerstone of treatment for patients having ST segment elevation myocardial infarctions (STEMI) by improving outcomes and preserving left ventricular function· There are in fact many large randomised clinical trials which support early thrombolysis and these can be found in the Fibrinolytic Therapy Trialists' (FTT) Collaborative Group publication from 1994. This document reinforces the importance of early reperfusion with 30 lives per 10000 being saved by thrombolysis given within 6 hours of presentation and 20 lives per 1000 saved if initiation is between 6 and 12 hours.

2. Pathophysiology of myocardial infarction

Acute myocardial infarction which is commonly known as a heart attack is the interruption of blood supply and therefore oxygen to heart muscle thereby potentially causing cell death or necrosis. This is usually due to the occlusion of the coronary artery lumen by clot called thrombus. This thrombus is formed by the rupture of unstable arteriosclerotic plaque which consists of white blood cells (mainly macrophages) which engulf lipids to form foam cells covered with a fibrous cap in the arterial wall. The plaque can rupture as a result of many factors including the mechanical shear stress from blood flow and flexion and tension of the fibrous causing it to be injured and thinned. Rupture exposes adhesion molecules in the sub-endothelium which form thrombus when exposed to flowing blood. This allows primary haemostasis to occur, resulting in platelet adhesion, platelet activation and aggregation forming thrombus. Thrombolytic drugs break down this thrombus thereby restoring blood flow and preventing further damage to myocardium. It is therefore obvious to see that the sooner myocardial infarction is diagnosed and the earlier thrombolysis can be given the greater the myocardial salvage.

3. Clinical indications

The indications for thrombolysis in myocardial infarction rely on eliciting a history of typical clinical symptoms (mainly but not exclusively chest pain) and diagnosing characteristic changes in the 12-lead electrocardiogram (ECG) which is a non-invasive means of recording the electrical activity of the heart over seconds using transthoracic electrodes. The prompt recognition of the characteristic symptoms and ECG changes are required to institute rapid reperfusion therapy through thrombolysis.

The main clinical symptom of acute myocardial infarction is central or left-sided chest pain which can be described as dull, squeezing or tightness. This is called angina pectoris. The pain most commonly radiates to the left arm but can radiate to the neck, jaw, epigastrium, back and the right side of the chest. The management of myocardial infarction also requires prompt relief of the ischaemic pain with oxygen, opiates and sublingual or intravenous nitrates which act through vasodilatation. Other symptoms are shortness of breath from left ventricular dysfunction and resultant pulmonary oedema due to myocardial ischaemia. The remaining symptoms are due to surges of catecholamines from sympathetic overdrive such as palpitations, nausea, vomiting, light-headedness, weakness, anxiety and excessive sweating termed diaphoresis. Loss of consciousness may also occur and is usually due to arrhythmia as a consequence of ischaemia or cerebral hypoperfusion due to poor left ventricular output and cardiogenic shock. Notably women tend to report more atypical symptoms and so when making a diagnosis clinicians should bare this in mind. To complicate matters further around one quarter of patients suffering an acute myocardial infarction do not have any symptoms at all. These 'silent' myocardial infarctions most commonly occur in the elderly and diabetic patients. This can cause problems when selecting out patients that are suitable for thrombolysis as the clinician would have to rely on the ECG criterion and any other relevant history that is available at that time.

Other scenarios where a history may be difficult to obtain are patients that are acutely breathless from pulmonary oedema or those that have been successfully resuscitated or are being resuscitated from cardiac arrest. In these situations if the ECG shows characteristic changes and the bleeding risk from chest compressions is felt to be low then an experienced clinician can make the decision to proceed with thrombolysis. In cardiac arrests with refractory ventricular fibrillation and a prior history of chest pain or ischaemic heart disease then also in these cases a decision may be taken to give thrombolysis.

4. Electrocardiogram criterion

The ECG criterion for thrombolysis are well validated and need to be met before initiation of therapy. As mentioned earlier the ECG is a recording of electrical activity as it spreads through the heart muscle. The ECG can be daunting in its interpretation and in itself a massive topic but here we focus specifically on the parts of the ECG that are relevant for diagnosing acute myocardial infarction suitable for thrombolysis.

Ventricular depolarisation and contraction are represented on the ECG by a waveform termed the QRS complex which is later followed by a smaller deflection termed the T wave which constitutes ventricular repolarisation and relaxation. In fact, repolarisation begins with the ST segment which connects the QRS complex to the T wave. The beginning of the ST segment is termed the J point.

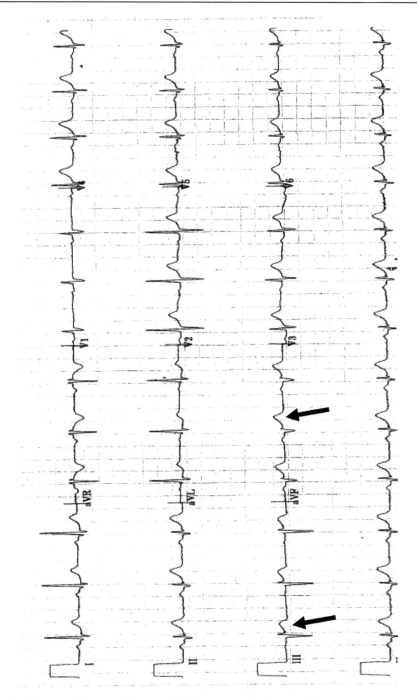

Fig. 1. An electrocardiogram showing ST elevation in leads III and AVF.

The criterion for thrombolysis refer to the QRS complex and ST segments and are as follows:

1. 1mm of ST segment elevation from the J point in at least 2 contiguous limb leads (I, II,III, AVF and AVL)
2. 2mm of ST segment elevation from the J point in at least 2 contiguous chest leads (any two of V1 to V6)

New onset left bundle branch block. This is recognised as characteristic deflections of the QRS complex and an increased width of greater than 120 milliseconds which is 3 small squares on the ECG when the recording speed is set to the usual 25mm/second.

The various limb leads and chest leads pick up electrical signals by literally overlying and 'pointing' towards various parts of the heart. Therefore ECG changes in certain leads represent ischaemia affecting certain territories or areas of heart muscle. ECG changes in leads I and AVR represent ischaemia in the anterior wall of the left ventricle while II, III, and aVF represent the inferior aspect of the heart. The V leads or chest leads show if the anterior-septal area is affected (V1-V4) and the late V leads signify infarction of the lateral wall of the ventricle. Leads I and AVL also represent the lateral territory of the heart. The criterion requires that these changes are in at least two contiguous leads because this is more likely to represent a significant area or 'territory' of myocardium. ST segment changes in a single lead are more likely to be due to other causes the most likely being normal variant due to an earlier repolarisation of the myocardium. Clinicians also need to bear in mind alternative diagnoses which could present with ST elevation by ECG. Acute pericarditis, which is a usually benign condition of pericardial inflammation, can present with ST elevation but typically the ST segment has a saddle-shaped appearance. The clinical symptoms may also mimic myocardial infarction but the classical description is of pain is different in that it is sharp and stabbing which varies with respiration and is also positional. Clinically the patient may also have an audible rub on auscultation using a stethoscope. This is a scratchy noise caused by the inflamed layers of pericardium rubbing against each other. The other condition in which ST elevation may be present is when the patient has an outpouching of the left ventricle termed an aneurysm. Again the ECG can have a more characteristic Clinicians should keep the possibility of these alternative diagnoses at the forefront of their minds to avoid misdiagnosis and therefore inappropriate administration of thrombolysis.

Other ECG changes that accompany ST elevation may also be present and aid the diagnosis of acute ST elevation myocardial infarction. The T waves may become hyperacute and lose their normal concavity. There may also be the presence of a pathological Q wave at the start of the QRS complex which is represented by a negative deflection of at least 1 small square on the ECG (40 milliseconds). This is said to represent infarcted non-viable myocardium. The other common abnormality which can accompany ST elevation is ST depression in reciprocal leads. Essentially, this means that leads looking at the opposite aspect of the heart show a mirror image of the leads showing ST elevation.

5. Contraindications for thrombolysis

Contraindications to thrombolysis in myocardial infarction can be separated into absolute and relative ones. Absolute contraindications are suspected dissecting aortic aneurysm, ischaemic stroke within 3 months (except if acute and within 3 hours of symptom onset when it is a treatment), intracranial neoplasm or arterio-venous malformation, active bleeding diathesis, uncontrolled hypertension (systolic>180mmHg or diastolic >100mmHg), significant closed-head trauma or facial trauma within 3 months.

Rigorous cardiopulmonary resuscitation or compressions of greater than 10 minutes duration is a relative contraindication to thrombolysis. Other scenarios which require precaution include active peptic ulceration, therapeutic anticoagulation with warfarin therapy, active menstruation, pregnancy, recent streptococcal infection of less than five days, controlled severe hypertension, haemorrhagic or diabetic retinopathy and invasive or surgical procedure in the preceding three weeks.

6. Evidence base for thrombolysis and alternative strategies

Initially, streptokinase infusion produced conflicting results until the (GISSI) trial in 1986, which validated streptokinase as an effective therapy and established a fixed regime for its use in acute myocardial infarction. As mentioned earlier the evidence supporting thrombolysis as opposed to not giving thrombolysis is outlined in the Fibrinolytic Therapy Trialists' (FTT) Collaborative Group publication from 1994. This combined the data from 9 trials and included a total of 58,600 patients. Here, the obvious survival advantage of thrombolysis in ST segment elevation in myocardial infarction and left bundle branch block was established. However, excess deaths were noted in the elderly and those thrombolysed after 12 hours of symptom onset. Most notably, it was clearly seen that the earlier thrombolysis was given the greater the benefit. The reason being that the earlier reperfusion is achieved the smaller the infarct size and the greater the myocardial salvage, which in turn has a significant impact on morbidity and mortality. This has led to targets for thrombolysis to be initiated within 20 to 30 minutes of arrival at hospital ("door to needle" time) and within 60 minutes of calling for help ("call to needle" time) across the UK and in Europe.

Primary percutaneous coronary intervention (PPCI) has evolved as an alternative emergency treatment for patients with STEMI. This is an invasive keyhole procedure which involves the passing of thin catheters from the femoral or radial arteries in to the aorta and then in to the openings of the coronary arteries to act as a conduit for various specialized equipment that can be used to treat the acute thrombus. The equipment used for this purpose are primarily clot extraction catheters termed extraction catheters, inflatable balloons and metal stents which act as a scaffold for keeping the arteries open. Although the number of patients receiving this treatment is steadily increasing because of the potential benefits, not all hospitals have the facilities to provide this therapy and so most patients in Europe still receive thrombolysis as initial management.

Once thrombolysis was established as a mode of treatment it was initially given in hospital by clinicians but with the extensive data that early thrombolysis yielded better outcomes there was a move towards pre-hospital thrombolysis (PHT). This involved emergency services giving thrombolysis at the scene on arrival to the patient.

Meta-analyses of RCTs show that PHT is superior to in-hospital thrombolysis (IHT) as it saves on average 30 minutes to 1 hour from the time between calling for medical help and initiation of thrombolysis. The time benefit is even more apparent where ambulance transport times are long. For this reason IHT is only reserved for those places that that do not offer PHT or PPCI. When PPCI is not available or offered around the clock then PHT becomes the treatment modality of choice to ensure the maximal myocardial salvage.

Comparison of Angioplasty and Prehospital Thrombolysis in Acute Myocardial Infarction (CAPTIM) compared PHT directly against PPCI. This showed that if thrombolysis was administered within 2 hours of symptom onset mortality data at 30 days strongly favoured this treatment over PPCI. However, after 2 hours the trend of outcomes reversed and PPCI became the treatment of choice. This was mirrored in the PRAGUE-2 trial which showed the benefits of IHT up to 3 hours.

In contrast to this the Primary Coronary Angioplasty vs. Thrombolysis (PCAT)-2 Trialists Collaborative Group meta-analysis looked at IHT versus an invasive strategy and showed that PPCI was superior to thrombolysis with lower mortality rates and risk of re-infarction. In the USA, guidelines favour the data on PHT over PPCI but also focus on the time factor with regards to reperfusion. They recommend that PHT should be given within 30 minutes after the arrival of emergency services at the scene and if this is not available and the patient is transferred to a hospital without PPCI facility then IHT should be given within 30 minutes of arrival at the centre (this is termed to door-to-needle time). If PPCI is offered in the hospital then actual disruption of the acute thrombus in the coronary artery should take place within 90 minutes (termed door-to-balloon time). European guidelines differ in that they prefer PPCI as the primary mode for reperfusion but with the several caveats. They stipulate that the procedure should be performed by a skilled operator in a high volume centre (operator performing more than 75 PCIs a year and the centre performing more than 200 PCIs) within 120 minutes of the first medical contact or within 90 minutes in patients receiving medical help within 2 hours from the onset of symptoms. If PPCI is not available then thrombolysis should be given within 3 hours of symptom onset with preference given to PHT over IHT.

7. Rescue PCI, routine PCI and facilitated PCI

When thrombolysis fails then rescue PCI should be considered. In the REACT trial patients that had not been successfully treated by thrombolysis after 90 minutes from initiating therapy (signified by less than 50% resolution of ST segment resolution by ECG) were randomized between conservative management, repeat thrombolysis and rescue PCI. This trial showed a clear benefit of the latter in all outcome data including 6 month mortality. Rescue PCI should therefore be offered to all patients within 12 hours of symptom onset. This may therefore involve patient transfer to a centre that offers a PCI service if not available at the hospital where the patient was thrombolysed or where they were taken after PHT. The exact definition of failed thrombolysis is controversial but the absence of chest pain is considered as misleading as opiates, analgesics and vasodilators may contribute to this. Generally accepted markers are taken as ST segment resolution of less than 50-70% and the time taken to assess whether thrombolysis has taken effect is between 45 and 90 minutes.

All patients should receive PCI subsequent to this, ideally within a period of 24 hours, but a benefit is even seen up to 30 days as evidenced by the CAPTIM trial. GRACIA-1, CARESS-in-AMI and the WEST trials all looked at PCI within a quicker time frame after thrombolysis and the overall results showed that this was comparable to PPCI outcomes when the post-thrombolysis PCI was performed within 24 hours. The very recent TRANSFER-AMI trial reinforced the benefits of a pharmaco-invasive strategy which compared PCI at 6 hours after thrombolysis with 'standard treatment' which involved thrombolysis with delayed angiography and PCI (after 24 hours). There was a statistically significant reduction in the primary endpoint of combined incidence of death, reinfarction, recurrent ischemia, new or worsening heart failure, or cardiogenic shock at 30 days for the pharmaco-invasive strategy (11% in the pharmaco-invasive arm vs. 17.2% in the standard treatment arm). There was also less recurrent ischaemia (0.2% vs. 2.1%) and reinfarction (3.4% vs. 5.7%) in the pharmaco-invasive strategy and fewer congestive heart failure (3.0% vs. 5.6%). On the other hand, there were more deaths and more patients experiencing cardiogenic shock in the pharmaco-invasive arm but these differences were not statistically significant. There were significantly more minor bleeding episodes in the combined strategy arm when compared to standard treatment but there was no difference in major bleeding. It is important to note that this pharmaco-invasive strategy is very different to thrombolysis followed by *immediate* PCI. This is called facilitated PCI and in fact has failed to shows clinical benefit and may in fact be harmful. The reason for this being that if PCI is performed too early then the thrombolytic administered is still active causing increased bleeding risk as well as resulting in more acute stent thrombosis (the potentially catastrophic blocking of a stent by thrombus within 24 hours of it being deployed) which is caused by the increased platelet activation and aggregation which accompanies thrombolytics.

The ideal setting for PHT in the USA involves an experienced physician being available to interpret the ECG by either being part of the Emergency Medical service team on the ambulance or being available to review a copy of a transmitted ECG. This has proved harder to achieve in Europe where more frequently, trained paramedics decide on whether the ECG meets criterion. Some UK studies have shown that this is safe and sometimes even better than the physician-assisted model due technological issues when transmitting the ECG or failure of mobile phones when trying to communicate to doctors from remote areas. However, in contrast a study in Finland has shown that having physicians on site for PHT is superior to paramedics alone. A checklist of contraindications should also be gone through prior to administration to ensure that the patient is not placed at increased risk of catastrophic bleeding. Therefore, this can also be used as a means of identifying those patients that are more suitable for PPCI.

8. Adjunctive therapies for thrombolysis

Aspirin is well established as an adjunctive therapy to thrombolysis and it is recommended that 150 to 325mg of chewable aspirin be given to the patient with thrombolysis. Clopidogrel is an oral, thienopyridine class antiplatelet agent which when given at a dose of 300 mg also provides prognostic benefit. The COMMIT-CCS-2 and CLARITY-TIMI 28 trials provided this evidence for adding clopidogrel to aspirin in patients undergoing fibrinolytic therapy.

It is recommended that unfractionated heparin, an intravenous anticoagulant is given intravenously with all of the thrombolytics to enhance clot dissolution and decrease the risk of re-occlusion. In vitro studies and animal models show discordant results regarding concomitant administration of heparin with thrombolysis suggesting that it may enhance, inhibit or have no effect. Hsia J et al.(1990) have shown that thrombolysis achieves faster lysis with greater vessel patency in combination with heparin (between 7 and 24 hours a patent vessel was found in 88% of those receiveing thrombolysis with heparin and aspirin vs. 52% in those treated with thrombolysis and aspirin alone). Unfortunately this does not translate into clinical outcome with a meta-analysis of the six trials by Muhaffey KW et al.

(1996) showing that there were similar rates of mortality and re-infarction before discharge. Despite this the general consensus from expert opinion is that heparin is beneficial in preventing re-occlusion and that it should be given as a bolus with all thrombolytics other than Streptokinase and then be given as a continuous IV infusion. With the advent of low molecular weight heparins (LMWHs) which only need once or twice daily subcutaneous administration without regular blood monitoring the continuous IV infusion of unfractionated heparin has been superseded by these newer anticoagulants. In fact there is evidence that the LMWH, Enoxaparin, appears superior to UFH in the EXTRACT-TIMI 25 trial when given during thrombolysis. In fact, patients under the age of 75 years can be given a 30 mg intravenous bolus followed by the subcutaneous dose every 12 hours. In practice this intravenous preparation LMWH is less widely available and UFH is more commonly given.

9. Thrombolytics used in clinical practice

9.1 Streptokinase

This was the first thrombolytic used in the treatment of STEMI and remains the cheapest and most commonly used. Two large trials were pivotal in demonstrating the efficacy of Streptokinase as a thrombolytic in myocardial infarction which reduces mortality when compared against placebo. The first of these was the GISSI trial mentioned earlier, published in 1986 and included 11,712 patients. This trial showed that at 21 days the mortality for patients treated with Streptokinase was 10.7% vs 13% for the placebo group which represented a statistically significant absolute reduction of 2.3% (risk ratio 0.81; 95% confidence ratio [CI] 0.72 to 0.9). The second trial, ISIS-2 trial included 17,187 patients and was published 2 years after GISSI in 1988. In this study, vascular mortality at 5 weeks was 9.2% in the streptokinase group and 12% in those treated with placebo which represented a statistically significant absolute reduction of 2.8%. Streptokinase is administered as an IV infusion over 1 hour. Streptokinase has a few side-effects which are namely low blood pressure termed hypotension, infrequent allergic reactions and sometimes although not commonly, anaphylaxis. Patients treated with streptokinase develop anti-streptococcal antibodies, which is why patients should only ever receive this drug once in a lifetime.

9.2 Alteplase

A meta-analysis of eight trials which compared alteplase with streptokinase found that there was no significant difference between the two drugs in terms of mortality up to 35 days. However, re-infarction rates were found to be in favour of alteplase but this was offset by a doubling in the risk of haemorrhagic stroke (odds ratio 2.13; 95% CI 1.04 to 4.36). In contrast to this, streptokinase was associated with a statistically significant higher risk of major bleeds than alteplase. However, the definitions of major bleeding varied between the trials and so it is difficult to judge the clinical significance of these findings.

9.3 Alteplase

Alteplase which is also known as recombinant human tissue plasminogen activator or rtPA can be delivered in a standard or accelerated regimen. The accelerated regimen, which is much more commonly used especially in PHT because of its ease of administration as it is delivered by an initial IV bolus injection. This is followed by only two IV infusions at 30 minutes and 60 minutes. The GUSTO-I trial was the only study in the meta-analysis mentioned above which looked at the more commonly used accelerated regimen rather than the standard regimen. This trial which included over 40000 patients was also the only trial to demonstrate superiority over different thrombolytics with an absolute reduction in mortality at 30 days of 1.0% (6.3% versus 7.3%; 95% CI 0.4% to 1.6%) in favour of accelerated alteplase when compared to streptokinase. However, this benefit was balanced by a statistically significantly higher incidence of haemorrhagic stroke (odds ratio 1.42; 95% CI 1.05 to 1.91). Using a combined outcome measure of mortality and disabling stroke, there was in fact a statistically significant absolute advantage of streptokinase over alteplase of 0.9%;p = 0.006). Interestingly, statistically significant rates of moderate bleeding or worse were lower in the alteplase group. Alteplase also fared better with regards to the common side effects experienced by streptokinase namely causing less allergic reactions, anaphylaxis, and sustained hypotension and these were also statistically significantly lower. Despite this a further meta-analysis of nine trials comparing standard alteplase with streptokinase, including the findings of GUSTO-I (i.e. accelerated alteplase), found no significant difference between the two drugs in terms of mortality up to 35 days (odds ratio 0.94; 95% CI 0.85 to 1.04).

9.4 Reteplase

This is the third most commonly used thrombolytic and one of the easiest to administer as it only involves two IV boluses administered 30 minutes apart. The INJECT study involving nearly 6000 patients compared reteplase to streptokinase. This study found an absolute difference in 35 day mortality of 0.5% (95% CI –1.98% to 0.96%) in favour of reteplase but this was not deemed as statistically significant. Similarly to alteplase, when a combined outcome measure using overall effects on mortality and disabling stroke is applied to the trial data then reteplase may in fact be inferior to streptokinase, as the trial also found a statistically significantly lower risk of haemorrhagic stroke in the streptokinase group (odds ratio 2.1; 95% CI 1.02 to 4.31). However, the trial also found that the in the reteplase group the rates of heart failure (23.6% vs 26.3%, p<0.05) and allergic reactions (1.1% vs 1.8%, p<0.05) were significantly lower. In one small study of 324 patients (RAPID-2), reteplase was compared to alteplase and this found that better vessel patency was achieved when coronary angiography was the endpoint. Subsequent to this the large GUSTO-III trial involving 15,059 was designed to test the clinical superiority of reteplase over accelerated alteplase. However, GUSTO-III found no statistically significant difference between the two drugs, in terms of survival or adverse effects but at 30 days mortality was 7.5% in the reteplase group and 7.2% in the accelerated alteplase group giving an absolute risk reduction of 0.23% in favour of accelerated alteplase (95% CI–1.10% to 0.66%). Therefore, reteplase cannot be considered as equivalent to accelerated alteplase.

9.5 Tenectaplase

This is the easiest of the thrombolytics to administer and only involves a single bolus. ASSENT-2 enrolled over 16,000 patients to compare tenecteplase and accelerated alteplase and found that 30-day mortality was the same in the tenecteplase group and the accelerated alteplase at 6.2% each, thereby showing equivalence in outcomes. In fact there was an absolute difference of 0.03% in favour of accelerated alteplase but this was not statistically significant (95% CI -0.55% to 0.61%). However, there was a small but statistically significant reduction in the incidence of bleeding with tenecteplase of 26.4% compared with 28.9% in the accelerated alteplase group. This resulted in fewer blood transfusions in the tenecteplase group (4.3% of patients compared with 5.5% in the accelerated alteplase group.

In summary, with regards to clinical effectiveness and mortality, standard alteplase and reteplase are as effective as streptokinase, and tenecteplase is as effective as accelerated alteplase. According to GUSTO-I, accelerated alteplase is believed to be superior to streptokinase and if this is the case then indirectly tenecteplase would also be considered to be superior to streptokinase (as tenectaplase was superior to accelerated alteplase in ASSENT-2). In practice, cost and availability is a significant issue with regards to what is ultimately used and also use may also go unchanged for long periods purely because of a specific thrombolytic having historical use in a certain area.

9.6 Other considerations

In the elderly, evidence suggests that thrombolysis provides a mortality benefit but that there is increased risk of adverse events and poor outcomes in those with advancing age. The main risk in the older age group is of intracerebral haemorrhage and this is why a clear benefit is seen for PPCI in patients above the age of 75 and in fact the benefit is maintained even when there are longer door-to-balloon times. Low body weight has also been found to be independently associated with increased mortality and morbidity. With regards to sex, it is accepted that there is no difference with regards to efficacy but studies have shown that for unknown reasons women are less likely to receive any type of reperfusion (thrombolysis or PPCI) than men. Anterior infarcts also seem to show an increased benefit with thrombolysis over other territories but this may simply reflect the increased baseline risk in this group. Overall, when clinicians are deciding who would benefit from thrombolysis it appears that patient selection is key and benefits should be balanced against any potential risks.

10. References

A comparison of reteplase with alteplase for acute myocardial infarction. The Global Use of Strategies to Open Occluded Coronary Arteries (GUSTO III) Investigators.. N Engl J Med 1997 Oct 16;337:1118-23

Armstrong P, WEST Steering Committee. A comparison of pharmacologic therapy with/without timely coronary intervention vs. primary percutaneous intervention early after ST-elevation myocardial infarction: the WEST (Which Early ST-elevation myocardial infarction Therapy) study. Eur Heart J 2006;27: 1530–1538.

Bode C, Smalling RW, Berg G, Burnett C, Lorch G, Kalbfleisch JM, Chernoff R, Christie LG, Feldman RL, Seals AA, Weaver WD. Randomized comparison of coronary thrombolysis achieved with double-bolus reteplase (recombinant plasminogen activator) and front-loaded, accelerated alteplase (recombinant tissue plasminogen activator) in patients with acute myocardial infarction. The RAPID II Investigators.. Circulation 1996;94:891-8

Cantor WJ, Fitchett D, Borgundvaag B, Heffernan M, Cohen EA, Morrison LJ, Ducas J, Langer A, Mehta S, Lazzam C, Schwartz B, Dzavik V, Goodman SG. Rationale and design of the Trial of Routine ANgioplasty and Stenting After Fibrinolysis to Enhance Reperfusion in Acute Myocardial Infarction (TRANSFER-AMI).. Am Heart J 2008;155:19-25

COMMIT collaborative group. Addition of Clopidrogel to aspirin in 45,852 patients with acute myocardial infarction: randomised placebo-controlled trial. *Lancet.* Nov 2005;366(9497):1607-21

Di Mario C, Dudek D, Piscione F, Savonitto S, Murena E, Dimopoulos K, Manari A, Gaspardone A, Ochala A, Zmudka K, Bolognese L, Steg PG, Flather M, on behalf of the CARESS-in-AMI investigatorsImmediate angioplasty versus standard therapy with rescue angioplasty after thrombolysis in the Combined Abciximab REteplase Stent Study in Acute Myocardial Infarction (CARESS-in-AMI): an open, prospective, randomised, multicentre trial. Lancet 2008;371:559–568.

"Effectiveness of intravenous thrombolytic treatment in acute myocardial infarction. Gruppo Italiano per lo Studio della Streptochinasi nell'Infarto Miocardico (GISSI)". Lancet 1 (8478): 397–402. 1986

Elliott M. Antman, M.D., David A. Morrow, M.D., M.P.H., Carolyn H. McCabe, B.S., Sabina A. Murphy, M.P.H., Mikhail Ruda, M.D., Zygmunt Sadowski, M.D., Andrzej Budaj, M.D., Jose L. López-Sendón, M.D., Sema Guneri, M.D., Frank Jiang, M.D., Ph.D., Harvey D. White, D.Sc., Keith A.A. Fox, M.B., Ch.B., and Eugene Braunwald, M.D. for the Enoxaparin versus Unfractionated Heparin with Fibrinolysis for ST-Elevation Myocardial Infarction (ExTRACT-TIMI 25) Investigators N Engl J Med 2006; 354:1477-1488April 6, 2006

Fernandez-Avile´s F, Alonso JJ, Castro-Beiras A, Vazquez N, Blanco J, Alonso-Briales J, Lopez-Mesa J, Fernandez-Vazquez F, Calvo I, Martinez-Elbal L, San Roman JA, Ramos B. Routine invasive strategy within 24 hours of thrombolysis versus ischaemia-guided conservative approach for acute myocardial infarction with ST-segment elevation (GRACIA-1): a randomised controlled trial. Lancet 2004;364:1045–1053.

Gershlick AH, Stephens-Lloyd A, Hughes S, Abrams KR, Stevens SE, Uren NG, de Belder A, Davis J, Pitt M, Banning A, Baumbach A, Shiu MF, Schofield P, Dawkins KD, Henderson RA, Oldroyd KG, Wilcox R; REACT Trial Investigators. Rescue angioplasty after failed thrombolytic therapy for acute myocardial infarction. N Engl J Med. 2005 Dec 29;353(26):2758-68.

Hsia J, Hamilton WP, Kleiman N, Roberts R, Chaitman BR, Ross AM. A comparison between heparin and low-dose aspirin as adjunctive therapy with tissue plasminogen activator for acute myocardial infarction. Heparin-Aspirin Reperfusion Trial (HART) Investigators. N Engl J Med. 1990; 323:1433-7.)

Muhaffey KW, Granger CG, Collins R, O'Connor CM, Ohman EM, Bleich SD, Col JJ, Califf RM. Overview of randomized trials of intravenous heparin in patients treated with thrombolytic therapy. Am J Cardiol 1996;77: 351-6.

Randomised, double-blind comparison of reteplase double-bolus administration with streptokinase in acute myocardial infarction (INJECT): trial to investigate equivalence. International Joint Efficacy Comparison of Thrombolytics. Lancet 1995;346:329-36

Sabatine MS, Cannon CP, Gibson CM, et al. Addition of clopidogrel to aspirin and fibrinolytic therapy for myocardial infarction with ST-segment elevation. *N Engl J Med*. Mar 2005;352(12):1179-89.

The GUSTO Investigators. An international randomized trial comparing four thrombolytic strategies for acute myocardial infarction. *N Engl J Med*. 1993;329:673-682.

Van De Werf F, Adgey J, Ardissino D, Armstrong PW, Aylward P, Barbash G, Betriu A, Binbrek AS, Califf R, Diaz R, Fanebust R, Fox K, Granger C, Heikkilä J, Husted S, Jansky P, Langer A, Lupi E, Maseri A, Meyer J, Mlczoch J, Mocceti D, Myburgh D, Oto A, Pao. Single-bolus tenecteplase compared with front-loaded alteplase in acute myocardial infarction: the ASSENT-2 double-blind randomised trial.. Lancet 1999 Aug 28;354:716-22

7

Prehospital Thrombolysis: It's All About Time

Raveen Naidoo and Nicholas Castle
Durban University of Technology
South Africa

1. Introduction

Prehospital emergency care personnel can play a crucial role in the identification and management of patients presenting with ST Elevation Myocardial Infarction (STEMI). Specifically, prehospital thrombolysis by emergency medical personnel such as paramedics/nurses/prehospital doctors has been identified as being a successful and safe approach for the provision of accelerating reperfusion strategies for acute STEMI. Moreover, prehospital thrombolysis has no added specific risks (arguably, it is safer as delayed thrombolysis increases the risk of myocardial rupture) as compared to inhospital thrombolysis; nor is it an obstacle for later percutaneous coronary intervention (PCI). This chapter will focus on the general management of STEMI, the potential benefits related to prehospital thrombolysis and alternative, adjunctive therapies and provide some useful hints to drug administration.

Prehospital thrombolysis is an established emergency treatment and has been classified as a Class IIa recommendation therapy for acute STEMI by the leading international cardiology societies like European Society of Cardiology (2008). Prehospital thrombolysis research is ongoing with a large multi-center trial currently recruiting patients in 112 locations worldwide – STREAM – Strategic Reperfusion Early After Myocardial Infarction. STREAM aims to evaluate, in a proof of concept approach, the outcome of prehospital patients presenting with acute STEMI within 3 hours of symptom onset. Following randomization, a treatment strategy of early (prehospital) tenecteplase and additional antiplatelet and antithrombin therapy followed by catheterization within 6-24 hours with timely coronary intervention as appropriate (or by rescue coronary intervention if required) compared to primary angioplasty. This intention to treat study will therefore place patients into two groups; Group A will receive primary PCI performed according to local standards and Group B will receive prehospital thrombolysis supported by optimal supportive adjunctive therapy (http://clinical trials.gov.show/NCT00623623).

2. Development of prehospital thrombolysis

The first published study of prehospital thrombolysis involved the intravenous administration of 750,000 units of streptokinase by physicians was undertaken in 1985. This study demonstrated that patients treated less than 1.5 hours after the onset of pain had a significantly higher ejection fraction (56±15 vs. 47±14 %; P<0.05), improved infarct-related regional ejection fraction (51±19 vs. 34±20 %; P<0.01) and a lower QRS score (5.6±4.9 vs.

8.6±5.5; P<0.01) than patients receiving treatment between 1.5 and 4 hours from the onset of pain. Patients in the prehospital arm of the study also had better-preserved left ventricular function than patients treated in the hospital. The study concluded that thrombolytic therapy with streptokinase is most effective when administered within 1.5 hours from onset of symptoms of acute myocardial infarction. Although this study produced positive results it lacked statistical power (due to small sample size) but it served to highlight the importance of timely thrombolysis (Koren et al., 1985).

Arguably, the Grampian Region Early Anistreplase Trial (GREAT) was the most influential prehospital thrombolysis based study. The aim of GREAT was to determine the time saved by thrombolysis when initiated at home by trained general practitioners (GPs) / family physicians as compared to thrombolysis inhospital. The GPs randomly assigned thrombolytic therapy to 311 patients with suspected acute myocardial infarction into two groups; prehospital thrombolysis and thrombolysis after arrival at the hospital. GPs selected patients on the basis of a history of chest pain from 20 minutes to 4 hours with treatment initiated within 6 hours from onset of pain. Patients in the prehospital treatment group received thrombolysis up to 130 minutes earlier than patients at hospital (101 vs 240 minutes from the onset of symptoms) with a 50% reduction in mortality in the prehospital group; 17 (10.4%) vs 32 (21.6%). The greatest saving of time was seen in the rural environment as well as in areas where there were significant inhospital treatment delays (Rawles, 1994). Importantly, during the GREAT study, prehospital thrombolysis was undertaken using a single bolus thrombolytic agent.

Patients enrolled in the GREAT study were followed up at five years where investigators noted 25% of the prehospital treatment group had died compared to 36% in the inhospital treatment group (Rawles, 1997). The GREAT study reconfirmed the negative impact of time delays by demonstrating that delaying thrombolysis by one hour increased the hazard ratio of death by 20%, with the equivalent loss of 43 lives per 1000 patients treated at five years. In a subset analysis of GREAT patients who met current ECG criteria for thrombolysis undertaken after 10 years, a 16% difference in mortality was maintained between the two groups (Rawles, 2003). The benefits seen in GREAT were significantly higher than those seen in any other thrombolysis study. The long-term mortality patterns has not been replicated in other long-term (inhospital) follow up studies, like ISIS-2 (1988) or GUSTO-1 (1993).

Treatment delays and the potential time savings of prehospital thrombolysis are key factors in the decision-making process around reperfusion with a meta-analysis by Morrison et al. (2000) of six randomized controlled trials clearly demonstrating the impact of the time savings to be achieved with prehospital treatment over inhospital treatment. Morrison et al. reported on all-cause hospital mortality as well as symptom to treatment time and adverse events. Although individual trials failed to demonstrate a statistically significant difference in all cause inhospital mortality; the meta-analysis involving 6434 patients showed a pooled benefit with prehospital thrombolysis. Morrison et al. demonstrated that prehospital thrombolysis saved approximately 60 minutes (p = 0.07) per patient compared to inhospital thrombolysis (104 versus 162 minutes) thereby reducing all-cause hospital mortality by 17%. If we consider the data from the five year follow up of the GREAT study, such time-savings can be extrapolated into significant numbers of lives saved.

Bjorklund et al. (2006) evaluated treatment delays and outcome in a large cohort of acute STEMI patients transported by ambulance who were either thrombolysed by paramedics in the prehospital environment or thrombolysed inhospital. Importantly, Björklund et al. utilized data from the Swedish / Register of Cardiac Intensive Care drawing data from 75 hospitals. Although register based data lacks the scientific controls seen within clinical trials, it is arguably more reflective of 'real life' clinical care. Following this study, Bjorklund et al. were able to conclude that prehospital thrombolysis by paramedics in ambulances was associated with reduced time to thrombolysis by almost 1 hour and reduced adjusted 1-year mortality by 30%.

Minimizing treatment delays in the administration of thrombolysis is key to optimizing patient outcomes. Although the LATE study (Becker, 1995) demonstrated clinical benefits of thrombolysis up to 12 hours, the greatest benefits were seen within 6 hours with the highest mortality reduction seen in those patients treated within the first 3 hours from onset of symptoms. The most commonly perceived post thrombolysis risks of stroke or major haemorrhage remain static regardless of when within the 12 hour period thrombolytic therapy is administered. However, the typically lethal complication of myocardial rupture exponentially increases after six hours. As demonstrated in the GREAT, WEST (Armstrong, 2006) and CAPTIM (Bonnefoy et al., 2009) studies prehospital thrombolysis is more likely to recruit patients within the first 6 hours of symptom onset; typically within the first 3 hours were the clinical benefit of treatment is at its highest.

These trails and others help to confirm the feasibility and safety of prehospital thrombolysis in a wide variety of circumstances and settings ranging from traditional ambulance services through to use by ship-based medical teams (cruise ships) and deployed military medicine. However, the choice between reperfusion strategies to manage acute STEMI remains a topic of interest. While it is agreed that primary PCI is the best strategy for acute STEMI it is still time sensitive and therefore needs to be performed in a timely manner and by experienced centres. This is not always achievable in developing countries, in rural health care settings or in remote medical facilities such as cruise ships.

3. Prehospital thrombolysis supported by early intervention

A number of mixed strategies for reperfusion have been studied; to include prehospital thrombolysis (full dose thrombolytic therapy) supported by rescue PCI for failed thrombolytic reperfusion (a hybrid reperfusion strategy) plus pre-discharge or symptom/ischaemia driven PCI, reduced dose thrombolysis supported by immediate PCI (facilitated PCI) and primary PCI. The ASSENT-4 PCI (2006) study demonstrated that facilitated thrombolysis, that is, thrombolysis immediately followed by PCI has been proven to be an unsuccessful intervention and will not be discussed further.

A hybrid reperfusion service involves implementing the best combination of reperfusion options to meet the unique requirements of the patient and typically involves early prehospital thrombolysis for those patients with the greatest benefit e.g. anterior STEMI presenting within 2-3 hours supported by rescue PCI and pre-discharge angioplasty with a system of primary PCI for the remaining patients. It must be re-iterated that primary PCI does still offer a superior treatment option when it is available in a timely manner.

The WEST trial investigated the use of a number of different reperfusion strategies, immediate prehospital thrombolysis plus usual inhospital care (excluding routine PCI), prehospital thrombolysis with compulsory rescue PCI for failed thrombolysis against primary PCI strategy. A key finding of the WEST study was a lower incidence of cardiogenic shock in patients who received thrombolysis early (within 3 hours) and the importance of prehospital triage/decisions for reperfusion with delays to definitive treatment being shorter when a decision was made in the prehospital setting. The WEST study also highlighted that thrombolysis used timeously remains an important treatment modality in the early management of acute STEMI.

The larger CAPTIM study used a similar design to the WEST study utilizing prehospital triage/decision to prehospital thrombolysis (this time supported by compulsory rescue PCI) with pre-discharge coronary intervention compared to primary PCI. The long term 5 year follow up of the CAPTIM study confirmed a significant reduction in mortality when thrombolysis was administered within 2 hours in the prehospital group when compared with primary angioplasty. The relationship between reperfusion strategy and the time from symptom onset on 1 year mortality was examined in a pooled analysis of patients from the CAPTIM and WEST studies. Mortality benefit was observed time (< 2 hours) (2.8% vs 6.9%, p = 0.021, hazard ratio 0.43, 95% CI 0.20-0.91) emphasizing that time from symptom onset was a key determinant when selecting the reperfusion strategy for acute STEMI (Westerhout et al., 2011). The optimal design of a hybrid reperfusion service is yet to be determined but the data from WEST and CAPTIM would support prehospital thrombolysis within the first 3 hours as along as all patients were delivered to a receiving hospital with interventional cardiology capability.

Prehospital thrombolysis can clearly be initiated earlier that inhospital thrombolysis or primary PCI and it can be performed with limited equipment. In fact, the same minimum equipment is required to perform prehospital thrombolysis as is required to identify prehospital patients requiring direct admission for primary PCI. Data from WEST (paramedic decision-makers), CAPTIM (doctor decision-makers) and projected findings from STREAM (paramedic/nurse/doctor decision-makers) are intended to inform the debate as to whether a hybrid reperfusion system is appropriate within developed countries. Regardless of the reperfusion strategy put into place, empowering the prehospital clinician is pivotal to success.

4. Education, training & equipment

The efficacy and safety of pre-hospital thrombolysis is dependent on several pre-requisites (Birkhead, 2004; Björklund et al., 2006; Mehta et al., 2002; Weaver, 1997; Welsh et al., 2006):

1. Prehospital personnel being trained to recognize symptoms and management of STEMI and its early complications (pain, ventricular fibrillation/ventricular tachycardia and bradycardic arrhythmias).
2. Diagnoses of STEMI using a 12 lead ECG with or without computer assistance for diagnosis and/or data transmission.
3. Intravenous access to be established and the administration of reperfusion therapy to be initiated within a treatment protocol / clinical guideline and supported by a thrombolysis checklist.

4. During transportation rhythm monitoring, availability of a defibrillator and advanced cardiac life support are mandatory
5. Pre-alerting receiving hospital of impending arrival of the patient supported by (if available) electronic transmission of the 12 lead ECG
6. Consultation for on-line support can support decision-making
7. On-going quality assurance

4.1 Education and training

The foundation for the practice of thrombolysis requires an understanding of anatomy and physiology of cardiovascular system and the pathophysiology of acute coronary syndromes. The complications of acute coronary syndromes / acute myocardial infarction must be covered as this will prepare the paramedic/nurse/prehospital doctor for complications that may arise during clinical practice. The ability to analyze a 12 lead ECG with a particular focus on recognition of AMI is required along with an understanding of thrombolytic therapy. An evidence based thrombolysis protocol which is subject to regular review is required taking into consideration the operational requirements for the practical implementation of the protocol. Classroom practice through the use of simulated clinical patient scenarios for stable angina, unstable angina, infarctions of the various territories including right ventricular infarction and scenarios where thrombolysis is contra-indicated will prepare and improve clinical practice. This theoretical and practical classroom education and training will need to be supported by clinical exposure within coronary care units and cardiac catheterization facilities.

4.2 Diagnosing acute STEMI

Van't Hof et al. (2006) demonstrated that prehospital diagnoses, triage and treatment in the ambulance is feasible in 95% of acute STEMI patients when undertaken by highly trained paramedics using a validated computerized ECG software. Prehospital decision-making can also be improved with the electronic transmission of an ECG although systems that support autonomous prehospital thrombolysis are well established and electronic data transmission can be problematic as they tend to rely on mobile telephone technology. The availability of prehospital 12 lead ECG capabilities serves to improve cardiac care in general and increased use of recording and subsequent interpretation of the 12 lead ECGs by prehospital clinicians improves overall confidence in using the prehospital ECG as a diagnostic tool. A particularly important aspect of the prehospital 12 lead ECG is that it is often obtained in the early phase of the patient's illness and becomes a useful ECG to compare against ECGs obtained later on in the patient's care.

The availability of diagnostic software and more importantly data transmission introduces an interesting concept for remote medical management of STEMI as the formal diagnosis of STEMI can be made by a distant clinician with the attending clinician acting primarily as a technician. This would involve the practical skills of cannulation, obtaining a 12 lead ECG and resuscitation skills (e.g. defibrillation) being undertaken by a junior clinician, but the decision to treat being made by a supervising clinician. This concept would expand the provision of prehospital thrombolysis whilst minimizing the education burden of the attending clinician and would be suitable for use in remote medical sites such as off shore oil platforms or small remote communities (e.g. Scottish Islands). Such a system is not dissimilar to the early use of defibrillation by paramedics where external supervision was required before defibrillation was performed.

5. Protocols, checklists & consent

5.1 Protocols

The use of clinicians empowered to make individual thrombolysis decisions removes the requirement for fixed protocols, however at the very least an evidence-based clinical guidelines for thrombolysis will be required. The availability of a clinical guideline or protocol will depend on the level of training provided to the prehospital clinician as guidelines support lateral thinking, whereas protocols tend to be more prescriptive.

The development of the thrombolysis protocol / guidelines needs to incorporate adjunctive therapy such as anti-thrombotic agents (e.g. heparin) and anti-platelets agents. This is an important aspect of patient care as to date none of the completed prehospital or inhospital thrombolysis studies have incorporated optimal anti-platelet and anti-thrombotic therapy. However, STREAM is currently utilizing the most up-to-date thrombolysis strategy.

5.2 Checklist

A thrombolysis checklist (Table 1), as part of a protocol / guideline, can support rapid decision-making whilst acting as a prompt to steps in the patient's management. However, care must be taken to ensure that the checklist is not overly restrictive as this can lead to under treatment of appropriate patients and careful consideration of the checklist layout can rapidly identify those patients where prehospital thrombolysis is deemed inappropriate e.g. advanced age (Castle et al., 2007a).

All contra-indications to thrombolysis need to be carefully considered and weighted. Often the type and number of contra-indications selected will reflect the risk adverse nature of the service delivering prehospital thrombolysis and, therefore, the list of contra-indications may change as the prehospital service becomes more established. It is now agreed that previous contra-indications such as prior cardiac compressions (Castle et al., 2007b; Cross et al., 1991) are no longer barriers to thrombolysis (in fact post cardiac arrest survivors with STEMI require urgent reperfusion with either PCI or hrombolysis); nor is diabetic retinopathy. (Mahaffey et al., 1997). Furthermore, complete heart block (CHB) is an indicator for rapid reperfusion therapy with thrombolysis being an accepted form of treatment as prompt reperfusion of the AV node (inferior STEMI with CHB) or intra-ventricular septum/Bundle of His (anterior STEMI with CHB) will resolve the arrhythmia thereby removing the need for a temporary pacing wire (Castle et al., 2007b) - the very reason typically quoted for with-holding thrombolytic therapy. All contra-indications to thrombolysis, with the exception of myocardial rupture as shown by the LATE Study (1993), are static/not affected by time whereas the benefit of thrombolysis is time dependent. Therefore, denying prehospital thrombolysis in a patient with STEMI based on one contra-indication only for the patient to be transferred to hospital for thrombolytic therapy to be administered will be counter-productive.

	Primary assessment: Can you confirm the following?	Yes	No
1	The patient is conscious and coherent, and able to understand that clot dissolving drugs will be used?		
2	The patient has symptoms that are characteristic of a heart attack (severe, continuous pain in a typical distribution of 15 minutes duration or more without remission)?		
3	The symptoms started less than 12 hours ago? NOTE: Consider "stuttering start" MI – many infarcts start this way.		
4	The pain built up over seconds and minutes rather than starting totally abruptly?		
5	Breathing does not influence the severity of the pain?		
6	The systolic blood pressure is more than 80mmHg and less than 180mmHg and that the diastolic is below 110mmHg despite treatment? i.e. Analgesia & GTN for blood pressure and fluid challenge / atropine for hypotension).		
7	The electrocardiogram ECG shows abnormal ST elevation of 2mm or more in at least 2 standard leads or in at least 2 adjacent precordial leads, not including V1? NOTE: ST elevation can sometimes be normal in V1 and V2.		
8	The QRS width is 0.16 seconds (4 small squares) or less, and that left bundle branch block is absent from the tracing? NOTE: RBBB is permitted only with qualifying ST elevation. LBBB = QRS 140 ms or greater; small narrow R wave in V1 & V2 with big S wave; tall upright monophasic R in standard Lead 1 and V6.		
	Secondary assessment (contra-indications): Can you confirm the following?	Yes	No
9	The patient is **not** likely to be pregnant, nor has delivered within the last 2 weeks?		
10	The patient has **not** had an active peptic ulcer within the last 6 months?		
11	The patient has **not** had a stroke of any sort within the last 12 months and does not have any permanent disability from a previous stroke?		
12	The patient has **no** diagnosed bleeding tendency, has had no recent blood loss (except normal menstruation) and is not taking warfarin (anticoagulant) therapy?		
13	The patient has **not** had any surgical operation, tooth extractions, significant trauma, or head injury within the last 4 weeks?		
14	The patient has **not** been recently treated for any other serious head or brain condition?		
15	The patient is **not** being treated for liver failure, renal failure, or any other severe systemic illness?		

Table 1. An example of a thrombolysis checklist

5.3 Consent

It is standard practice to obtain consent from the patient for thrombolytic therapy. The complications from thrombolysis are well documented. The patient will need to be appraised of the risks in undergoing thrombolysis. A standard statement that is simple, clear and concise is used in most established prehospital settings. An example of such a statement is as follows (Table 2):

However, it remains arguable whether a patient in pain or post opiate administration is in a position to give informed consent. It, therefore, falls to the attending clinician to ensure that they are working in the patient's best interest.

Initial Consent

"It is likely that you are having a heart attack and the best treatment available to you is a clot dissolving drug called (*specify agent*). The quicker you receive this drug, the lower the risks of a heart attack-which is why Doctors recommend that the treatment is started as soon as possible. These drugs can cause serious side effects in a small minority of patients which I can explain to you in more detail if you so wish, but the risks attached to this treatment are very much less than the likely benefit. Would you like me to give you the injection or would you prefer to have more details?'

I hereby consent to the treatment:

_____   _____/_____   _____

Name of patient   Date / Time   Signature / Thumbprint

In the unlikely event that the patients do want more information they should be given the following information:

Further information

"Treatment at this stage saves the lives of about 1 in every 25 treated. But it can sometimes cause serious bleeding. The biggest risk is stroke which affects about 1 patient in every 200 treated. Some patients also have allergic and other effects that do not usually cause any major problems. Would you like me to give you the injection?"

Table 2. An example of consent

6. Drugs

6.1 Thrombolytic agents

There are a number of thrombolytic agents available, however Tenecteplase (TNK) is the only single-use bolus agent available making it the most suitable for prehospital use. Despite this, the ideal thrombolytic agent currently does not exist.

The characteristics of an "ideal thrombolytic agent" are as follows:

- Rapid reperfusion (15 - 30 minute)
- 100% efficacy at achieving 100% TIMI 3 in 30 minutes
- Administered as a single intravenous bolus
- Lower incidences of intracranial haemorrhage
- Lower incidences of systemic bleeding and other complications.
- Specific for recent thrombi
- Lower incidences for re-occlusion
- Long-term sustained patency
- No antigenicity
- No negative interaction with adjunctive therapy
- Affordable

The GUSTO trial (1993) demonstrated the superiority of the accelerated regimen of tissue plasminogen activator (tPA, Alteplase) over Streptokinase (STK), however, this came at a price of slightly greater risk of intracranial haemorrhage especially in female patients over the age of 75 years. However, stroke after thrombolysis is a known risk and in the GUSTO trial the stroke rate with STK was 1.19% compared to 1.55% with tPA (Gore et al., 1995). The issue of stroke is an important consideration as denying thrombolysis does not decrease the stroke rate as STEMI is an independent risk factor for stroke - unrelated to thrombolysis primarily due to the higher incidence of atrial fibrillation (AF) and poor left ventricular (LV) function caused by STEMI. Therefore, early treatment of STEMI with reperfusion that reduces the incidence of AF and LV dysfunction is an important aspect of stroke and morbidity reduction.

Single bolus TNK is now the most widely used thrombolytic agent in the developed world partly due to its improved efficacy but also because of ease of administration and variable dosing. TNK and Alteplase are equivalent in regard to 30 day mortality, but non-cerebral bleeding and blood transfusions are less with TNK.

The dose of TNK is weight adjusted and administered in a single bolus over 5 seconds as compared to 90 minutes of variable rate infusion with tPA or a 30 - 60 minute infusion of STK. Although a 30 minute regime for STK exists, it is associated with an increased risk of hypotension but by slowing the infusion rate of STK, the incidence of hypotension tends to decrease. Reteplase is a more fibrin specific agent administered as a 10 unit twin bolus given 30 minutes apart. However, the time sensitive nature of the twin bolus administration of Reteplase can be problematic. Reteplase is equivalent with reduction in mortality and hemorrhage rates achieved with Alteplase.

The major benefit of the bolus agents lies in the ease of administration and in the simplified dosing regimen that reduces the risk of dosing errors. However, the cost of TNK and its manufacturer's recommendation for use up to 6 hours makes the cheaper STK a more practical drug of choice for use in the developing world as for each patient treated with TNK five patients could be treated with STK (Table 3) (BNF, 2011). Its use as a prehospital thrombolytic is worth consideration, particularly in static remote health care settings, although its requirement for an infusion plus the incidence of hypotension makes it more labour intensive.

	Streptokinase (STK)	Alteplase (tPA)	Reteplase (rtPA)	Tenecteplase (TNK)
Fibrin selective	No	Yes	Yes	Yes
Plasminogen binding	Indirect	Direct	Direct	Direct
Duration of infusion (minutes)	60	90	10 + 10	5-10 seconds
Half life (minutes)	23	<5	13-16	20
Fibrinogen breakdown	4+	1-2+	Not known	>tPA
Early heparin	Yes	Yes	Yes	Yes
Hypotension	Yes	No	No	No
Allergic reactions	Yes	No	No	No
Approximate cost/dose	£83.44/1.5 MU	£600/100 mg	£627.27/20 unit kit	£502.25/50 mg
TIMI reflow grade 3 at 90 min	32	45-54	60	>tPA
Recommended use	Up to 12 hours	Up to 12 hours	Up to 12 hours	Up to 6 hours (typically used up to 12 hours)

Table 3. Characteristics of commonly used thrombolytic agents. Adapted from Opie (2009).

There are two key considerations for the use of STK in the prehospital environment. The first is duration of infusion and second the requirement for an expensive infusion pump. Although an infusion pump offers better control of drug delivery, this is less of an issue with STK as the delivery of STK is less time sensitive when compared to tPA. In static medical care environments (e.g. remote medical center) the infusion can be completed before hospital transfer as STK can be safely delivered without an infusion pump using either a small intravenous bag (100/250ml 0.9% saline) or a pediatric burette supported by close clinician supervision. The use of a pediatric burette or a 100/250ml bag of saline is not an option for administration during ambulance transfer as the low ceilings in ambulances lack the height to ensure fluid flow and this is further aggravated by ambulance movement. Novel techniques involving the use of low cost drip counters (that restrict flow through an administration set) supported by a pressure infusion bag to maintain a constant pressure through the drip counter is feasible but as yet, is unproven.

The second consideration is the much higher incidence of hypotension and bradycardia. This is due to the release of bradykinin and not as commonly thought as an allergic reaction (although anaphylaxis is more common with STK, it remains rare). Therefore, the treatment of hypotension consists of slowing or stopping the infusion and the administration of a 250-500ml crystalloid bolus. The routine use of intravenous steroids and anti-histamines offers no clinical benefit and in the case of intravenous steroids, it may adversely affect patient outcome by affecting myocardial scar tissue formation, thereby potentially increasing the risk of myocardial rupture.

Streptokinase	Tenecteplase
1.5 mega units over 30-60 minutes (requires an infusion pump)	Single weight adjusted bolus
Aspirin 300mg	Aspirin 300mg
Clopidogrel age adjusted (75-300mg)	Clopidogrel age adjusted (75-300mg)
No heparin (local policy my vary)	Weight adjusted heparin bolus followed by infusion or weight adjusted subcutaneous injection of heparin: 4000 unfractionated heparin bolus followed by infusion (an infusion pump is mandatory) Age adjusted enoxaparin.
Bradycardia (common) reversed by atropine	Bradycardia (less common than STK) reversed by atropine
High risk of drug induced hypotension responsive to fluid challenge stopping/slowing infusion	No specific drug induced hypotension
Labour intensive	Not labour intensive
Affordable (if no infusion pump used)	Expensive

Table 4. Comparison of a STK and TNK treatment regime

6.2 Adjunctive drug treatment

6.2.1 Oxygen

Oxygen is commonly administered during the management of patients during thrombolysis. Its routine use in patient with pulse oximetry above 95% has been questioned primarily due to the possibility of vasoconstriction and limited evidence of benefit (O'Driscoll, 2008). Oxygen remains an important adjunctive therapy in the presence of left ventricular failure although it is better provided as part of continuous positive airway pressure. Oxygen should routinely be administered in the presence of arrhythmias (e.g. ventricular tachycardia) (Neumar, 2010), hypotension/hypo-perfusion and any post cardiac arrest.

6.2.2 Analgesia

Analgesia is a priority therapy in the management of STEMI and intravenous opiates (morphine, diamorphine or fentanyl) offer the most effective analgesia although the legal framework for administration of these drugs can be problematic resulting in drugs such as Tramadol or Nubain being used if legal barriers to opiates do exist. The use of inhaled nitrous oxide (Entonox™) remains a useful supplementary analgesic (or primary analgesic if prehospital opiates are not available) providing both supplementary oxygen and analgesia and the use of Pentrane (common in Australia) is also a useful inhaled analgesic allowing higher percentage of inhaled oxygen if required. Thrombolysis also represents effective analgesia as the restoration of myocardial blood flow results in pain relief reflecting successful reperfusion.

Non-pharmacological interventions (re-assurance, calm professional mannerism of the care provider) are important aspects of pain relief. The use of rapid road transfer with lights and sirens may induce greater patient anxiety (as well as the risk of road traffic collision). If prehospital thrombolysis has been administered (with appropriate adjunctive therapy) there is little to be gain from rapid transfer to hospital.

6.2.3 Nitrates

Although there is no survival benefit to be gained from nitroglycerin it remains a common early therapy primarily providing analgesia. Nitroglycerin (0.4mg) is typically administered sublingually although intravenous nitrates are also used to manage on-going ischaemic chest discomfort, control of hypertension and for the management of pulmonary oedema (nitrates are a Class I recommendation for left ventricular failure). Nitrates should not be administered to patients who have received phosphodiesterase inhibitor within 24 to 48 hours and should be administered with care in patients with suspected right ventricular infarction as they may induce marked hypotension. Despite this, nitrates are very safe drugs for use by prehospital clinicians and it must be remembered that known cardiac patients may have already treated themselves with varying doses of nitrates prior to the arrival of the prehospital clinician.

6.2.4 Antiplatelet agents

Antiplatelets are vital in the management of all acute coronary syndromes (unstable angina, non-STEMI and STEMI). Within the context of STEMI management anti-platelet therapy is as important as thrombolytic therapy. This is because the intra-coronary thrombus responsible for re-infarction tends to be platelet rich and thrombolysis may raise the possibility of thrombolytic-induced platelet aggregation (Keeley et al., 2006).

6.2.4.1 Aspirin

All patients with suspected acute coronary syndrome (unstable angina, non-STEMI and acute STEMI), should be considered for prehospital aspirin treatment as there are relatively few contra-indications to a single dose of aspirin (Class I recommendation). Despite this, aspirin is often withheld either due to concerns over allergy, adverse drug interactions (e.g. Warfarin), confusion due to chronic ongoing use of aspirin or uncertainty of diagnosis. Typically unless a patient has a known documented allergic reaction (not just gastric irritation) to aspirin or is actively bleeding from a gastrointestinal tract ulcer, aspirin at the 300mg dose should be given. The choice of 300mg is typically the dose of a single aspirin with the administration being initiated as early as possible with consideration being given to emergency call takers being empowered to recommend aspirin before the arrival of emergency personnel (Class IIb recommendation).

The benefit of aspirin was established in the ISIS 2 trial (1988) where 162.5 mg aspirin resulted in 25 lives saved per 1000 patients primarily by reducing the incidence of re-infarctions (10 non-fatal re-infarctions per 1000) as well as preventing 3 non-fatal strokes per 1000 patients. The results from ISIS 2 highlighted that the effectiveness of aspirin alone was nearly as effective as STK without aspirin (23% v 25% odds reduction of death) and that by combining aspirin with STK, the magnitude of benefit was highly significant (42% odds reduction of death). It is noteworthy that aspirin administration during the ISIS 2 trial was anytime within the first 24 hours but a meta-analysis by Freimark et al. (2002) demonstrated that early aspirin administration (before thrombolysis) was an independent factor in patient survival at 1 year (5% vs 11% survived with early aspirin; odds ratio 0.41; 95% CI 0.21-0.74).

The benefits of aspirin for acute STEMI are attributed to its inhibition cyclo-oxygenase dependent platelet activation. The administration of an initial dose of 160-300mg aspirin ideally non-enteric coated formulation chewed is a Class I recommendation for acute STEMI. Intravenous or rectal aspirin are also acceptable routes of administration.

Although over-treatment of patients or the administration of an unnecessary treatment cannot be endorsed, the benefits of early use of aspirin in any patient with symptoms suspected of a STEMI (or other acute coronary syndrome) is such that the potential of over-treatment of patients is arguably worth the risk, especially when comparing the maximum acute anti-platelet dose of aspirin (300mg) to the analgesic dose of aspirin of 600-900mg.

6.2.4.2 Clopidogrel

Clopidogrel is a potent platelet inhibitor and the anti-platelet benefits of clopidogrel in combination with aspirin is to reduce ischaemic events in non ST-elevation acute coronary syndromes (Yusuf et al., 2001) and in patients undergoing percutaneous coronary intervention - PCI CLARITY (2005). The COMMIT-CCS 2 (2005) trial involving more than 45 000 patients (many post thrombolysis) demonstrated that administration of Clopidogrel (75mg daily) with aspirin and standard treatment safely reduced mortality and major vascular events. In the CLARITY-TIMI 28 Trial (2006), patients 75 years and younger with acute STEMI received thrombolysis supported by a loading dose of 00mg Clopidogrel followed by 75mg once daily and either low molecular weight heparin (LMWH) or unfractionated heparin (UFH). The combination of dual anti-platelet therapy (aspirin/clopidogrel) with thrombolytic treatment demonstrated more favorable angiographic patency of the infarct related artery and a reduction in mortality. A major contributor to mortality reduction was the reduction in the re-infarction rate in those patients receiving dual anti-platelet therapy. This was without an associated increase in the rate of bleeding.

The importance of improved patency and lower incidence of re-infarction was confirmed in the ECG CLARITY-TIMI 28 Study (2006) where the use of clopidogrel was shown to improve late coronary patency and clinical outcomes in those patients who achieve ST-segment resolution by preventing re-occlusion of open arteries rather than by facilitating early reperfusion. The administration of 300mg loading dose of clopidogrel in association with thrombolysis to patients less than 75 years of age is a Class IIa recommendation and it is common practice to adjust the dose in the over 75 year old patients to 75mg based on the COMMIT data.

Newer oral antiplatelets such Prasugrel and Ticagrelor are now available with potentially improved antiplatelet as Ticagrelor produces a more profound and consistent antiplatelet effect than clopidogrel (Wallentin et al., 2003), but as yet to be studied in conjunction with thrombolytic therapy.

6.2.5 Anticoagulants

Heparin is considered to be effective and is routinely given as an adjunct for PCI and thrombolytic therapy although it is commonly withheld in the first 24 hours in those patients receiving STK. The role of heparin is primarily to reduce re-infarction but the combination of dual anti-platelet therapy, thrombolysis and heparin may increase the risk of bleeding. The American Heart Association guidelines call for careful weight based dosing of heparin with thrombolytic therapy in STEMI (Antman et al., 2008).

The timing of heparin therapy when using fibrin specific thrombolytic agents (tPA, reteplase and TNK) is an important aspect of patient management. In an observational study of the United Kingdom (UK) national registry the frequency of re-infarction during hospital admission after thrombolytic treatment of 35, 356 STEMI patients during 2005–2006 was analyzed. Re-infarction rates with inhospital treatment were similar for reteplase (6.5%) and TNK (6.4%) but were higher for those patients treated by paramedics in the community. When the interval from prehospital treatment to hospital arrival was greater than 30 minutes re-infarction rates were 12.5% for reteplase, and 11.4% for TNK. For intervals shorter than 30 minutes the re-infarction rates were significantly greater for TNK (9.3% than reteplase (4.2%). Overall, re-infarction rates were higher after prehospital treatment with TNK than reteplase (9.6% vs 6.6%, p=0.005).

The differences in re-infarction rates were considered to be primarily due to the different uses of adjunctive anti-thrombotic therapy as UK paramedic thrombolysis protocols only allowed a single bolus dose of heparin prior to thrombolysis but did not allow for ongoing heparinization until arrival inhospital as compared to inhospital practice which resulted in either an infusion of UFH (800-1000 IU per hour adjusted to aPTT) or weight adjusted LMWH. It was also noted that on arrival at hospital there was often a delay in the commencement of heparin therapy, either due to confusion about the prehospital protocol or other time related pressures. In addition, clopidogrel was commonly administered early in association with inhospital thrombolysis but only after arrival at hospital for those patients receiving prehospital thrombolysis (Horne et al., 2009). This may also have been a confounding factor as Keeley (2006) noted that thrombolysis induced platelet aggregation was a possible cause of re-infarction following thrombolysis.

UFH has long been regarded as the anti-thrombotic agent of choice in the adjunctive treatment of patients with STEMI until the introduction of enoxaparin. The ASSENT-3 PLUS Trial (2003) evaluated the feasibility, efficacy and safety of prehospital enoxaparin or UFH with tenecteplase. There was a reduction in the composite of 30 day mortality, inhospital re-infarction or inhospital refractory ischemia in the enoxaparin group (14.2% vs 17.4%., p = 0.08). However, there was a tendency towards higher rates of intracranial haemorrhage (ICH) and major bleeding in the enoxaparin group. The risk for ICH and major bleeding was mainly confined to patients > patients over 75 years. It must be noted that in ASSENT-3 PLUS, the dose of enoxaparin was not weight adjusted. The safety concern of enoxaparin among elderly patients was addressed by the ExTRACT-TIMI-25 Trial (2005) that randomized more than 20 000 thrombolysed patients to receive either enoxaparin or UFH. The ExTRACT-TIMI 25 study was significantly changed from the ASSENT 3 study with patients > to greater than 75 years of age not receiving the IV bolus of enoxaparin as well as receiving a reduced dose of subcutaneous enoxaparin (75%) with a maximum ceiling dose of subcutaneous enoxaparin for the patients under 75 being set at 100mg and 75mg for the over 75 age group. The primary endpoint of this study was all cause mortality or non-fatal reinfarction at 30 days. Treatment with enoxaparin was found to be superior to UFH but was associated with an increase with major bleeding episodes. A telephone follow up at 1 year showed a sustained reduction in mortality or re-infarction when using the enoxaparin strategy (Morrow et al., 2010). Data from a meta-analysis from 12 earlier trials involving more than 49 000 patients support these results (Murphy et al., 2007). Enoxaparin is administered as an initial dose of 30mg intravenous bolus, followed by 1mg/kg subcutaneously within 15 minutes and is a Class I recommendation.

The likely reason for both the reduction in re-infarctions but also the increased risk of bleeding associated with enoxaparin is that enoxaparin (in fact all LMWHs) provide more predictable anticoagulation. Whereas UFH is both dose and person sensitive typically requiring frequent dose changes as dictated by aPTT and commonly results in either under or over anti-coagulation.

Enoxaparin offers a number of operational benefits for use with prehospital thrombolysis; primarily the absence of an infusion pump that is required when administering an infusion of UFH. Two single 100mg dose syringes of enoxaparin is adequate to support prehospital thrombolysis with one syringe being used for the 30mg IV dose followed by subsequent subcutaneous dose (the maximum subcutaneous dose of enoxaparin remains 100mg). The intravenous dose of enoxaparin can be simply administered by decanting all of a 100mg dose of enoxaparin into a 10ml syringe and then diluting with water for injection to a total volume of 10mls thereby providing 10mg enoxaparin per ml. A multiple use vial of enoxaparin for IV administration is also available.

6.2.6 Steroids and antihistamines

The routine administration of steroids and antihistamines to prevent hypotension/bradycardia especially in association with Streptokinase complicates the administration process and is unlikely to prevent hypotension as the cause of Streptokinase induced hypotension is primarily due to speed of administration (Lew et al., 1985; Tatu-Chiţoiu et al., 2004) and the action of bradykinin activated by Streptokinase (Hoffmeister et al., 1998).

Tatu-Chiţoiu et al (2004) noted that the incidences of hypotension occurred in nearly half of all patients treated with Streptokinase but it did not adversely affect patient outcome whereas the prophylactic use if steroids is linked with an increased risk of myocardial rupture (Mannisi et al., 1987) and is not recommended by the leading international cardiology societies (Van de Werf et al., 2008).

7. Support systems

Studies have clearly demonstrated that thrombolytic therapy can be safely administered in the prehospital environment by doctors, paramedics and nurses. The most effective system will depend on population demographics, geographical factors, the structure and financial resources of the emergency medical services. Regardless of who undertakes thrombolysis, the personnel need to be capable of rapid diagnosis, early risk stratification, minimal treatment delay and rapid administration of a thrombolytic agent. EMS systems vary throughout the world. In 75% of Europe thrombolysis is undertaken by emergency physicians while in many other settings like United Kingdom, Australia and United States of America, it is undertaken by paramedics. In most countries, the use of non-doctors in the prehospital environment seems to be the most practical and cost effective option.

The practice of paramedic thrombolysis may be undertaken independently or under direct supervision depending on the local emergency medical system. A system of consultation and 12-lead ECG transmission with CCU nurses/a senior paramedic/specialist clinician experienced in STEMI management is highly recommended at the initial implementation of thrombolysis and for on-going clinical support in difficult cases (Liem et al., 2007; McLean et al., 2008). Furthermore, paramedics can also fast track acute STEMI patients to CCU by by-passing the emergency department as well as by-passing local hospitals to deliver the patient to a hospital with an on-site catheter laboratory for either rescue angioplasty or pre-discharge angioplasty. These strategies have demonstrated reductions in door-to-balloon time and mortality (Afolabi et al., 2007; Bång et al., 2008; Le May et al., 2006).

The transmission of 12-lead ECG may be challenging and is dependent of the use of cellular technology which may result in the inability to transmit the ECG due to poor coverage or drop zones. The transmission of the ECG may involve the pairing of cellular phones and ECG machines therefore will need to be tested and practiced to prevent user error.

8. Quality assurance

An on-going continuous professional development programme which incorporates quality improvement measures obtained by on-going monitoring of prehospital thrombolysis via clinical audit and feedback should be mandatory for continued safe prehospital thrombolysis and staff development. A clinical review team incorporating all role players would need to meet regularly to appraise all cases of prehospital thrombolysis. In settings where the frequency of the performance of thrombolysis is low, an on-going programme of refresher training is essential to maintain skill competence. External surveillance registries like MINAP and the Swiss registries provide valuable information on trends in management of acute STEMI and should be used to guide treatment timeframes and clinical outcomes.

9. Other uses for prehospital thrombolysis

Prehospital thrombolysis is primarily aimed at the treatment of patients with symptoms and ECG diagnosis of STEMI. Although this will remain the mainstay of the use of thrombolytic therapy, thrombolysis is also used in the treatment of other clinical emergencies.

9.1 Stroke

Although stroke thrombolysis is not suitable for initiation in the community due to the need for a CT scan and in a small subset of patients an MRI, the early identification of patients with a possible stroke is vital. This has required a change in emphasis within emergency departments and ambulance services where an acute stroke has now been identified as a time-sensitive clinical emergency. The UK has just completed a mass TV awareness campaign for the recognition of stroke, building on the brain attack model developed in

America. Prehospital clinicians are, therefore, pivotal in the early identification of suspected stroke patients typically using the **F**ast, **A**rm, **S**peech, **T**est (FAST) supported by pre-arrival alerts to hospitals equipped to deliver stroke thrombolysis (with 3-4 hours of onset of symptoms).

9.2 Cardiopulmonary resuscitation (CPR)

The use of thrombolysis during resuscitation is also a potential treatment option but the routine administration of thrombolysis during cardiac arrest management is not endorsed (Class III recommendation). However, its use to treat a confirmed or suspected massive pulmonary embolism or STEMI should be considered on a case-per-case bases (Class IIa recommendation) (Neumar, 2010). Confirmation of diagnosis remains challenging but is primarily based on clinical history supported by clinical suspicion although the use of bedside ECHO for the diagnosis of massive pulmonary embolism is worth consideration (typically to look at the right ventricle) but the expertise for this is limited in the prehospital environment.

Following the administration of thrombolytic therapy, during CPR, the period of resuscitation should be extended to a minimum of 60 minutes (Neumar, 2010) and this protracted period of resuscitation is an important consideration when initiating thrombolytic therapy. The administration of thrombolysis during resuscitation does not replace the need for effective compressions and supportive ventilation but represents a targeted treatment for a small subset of patients.

10. Conclusion

Prehospital thrombolysis offers two unique clinical pathways for the patient presenting with STEMI. Prehospital thrombolysis can be the preferred reperfusion strategy in developing countries or countries without rapid access to primary angioplasty facilities or can provide ultra-early reperfusion as part of a hybrid reperfusion service. Key to the success of any prehospital service is the recruitment and training of appropriately qualified personnel although in remote areas the use of telemedicine and electronic data transmission can support the administration of thrombolysis by junior clinicians. Although thrombolysis offers significant patient benefits, it needs to be appropriately delivered and supported by adjunctive therapy which should include dual anti-platelet therapy for all patients supported by heparin (ideally LMWH) as appropriate.

11. References

Afolabi, B. A., G. M. Novaro, S. L. Pinski, K. R. Fromkin and H. S. Bush (2007). Use of the prehospital ECG improves door-to-balloon times in ST segment elevation myocardial infarction irrespective of time of day or day of week. *Emergency Medicine Journal*, Vol. 24,No. (8), pp. 588-591.

Antman, E. M., M. Hand, P. W. Armstrong, E. R. Bates, L. A. Green, L. K. Halasyamani, J. S. Hochman, H. M. Krumholz, G. A. Lamas, C. J. Mullany, D. L. Pearle, M. A. Sloan and S. C. Smith, Jr. (2008). 2007 Focused Update of the ACC/AHA2004 Guidelines for the Management of Patients With ST-Elevation Myocardial Infarction: A Report of the American College of Cardiology/American Heart Association Task Force on

Practice Guidelines Developed in Collaboration With the Canadian Cardiovascular Society Endorsed by the American Academy of Family Physicians. *Journal of American College of Cardiology*, Vol. 51,No. (2), pp. 210-247.

Antman, E. M., D. A. Morrow, C. H. McCabe, F. Jiang, H. D. White, K. A. A. Fox, D. Sharma, P. Chew and E. Braunwald (2005). Enoxaparin versus unfractionated heparin as antithrombin therapy in patients receiving fibrinolysis for ST-elevation myocardial infarction: Design and rationale for the Enoxaparin and Thrombolysis Reperfusion for Acute Myocardial Infarction Treatment-Thrombolysis In Myocardial Infarction study 25 (ExTRACT-TIMI 25). *American Heart Journal*, Vol. 149,No. (2), pp. 217-226.

Armstrong, P. W. (2006). A comparison of pharmacologic therapy with/without timely coronary intervention vs. primary percutaneous intervention early after ST-elevation myocardial infarction: the WEST (Which Early ST-elevation myocardial infarction Therapy) study. *European Heart Journal*, Vol. 27,No. (13), pp. 1530-1538.

Bång, A., L. Grip, J. Herlitz, S. Kihlgren, T. Karlsson, K. Caidahl and M. Hartford (2008). Lower mortality after prehospital recognition and treatment followed by fast tracking to coronary care compared with admittance via emergency department in patients with ST-elevation myocardial infarction. *International Journal of Cardiology*, Vol. 129,No. (3), pp. 325.

Becker, R. C., Charlesworth, A., Wilcox, R.G., Hamptom, J., Skene, A., Gore, J.M., Topol, E.J. (1995). Cardiac Rupture Associated with Thrombolytic Therapy: Impact of time to Treatrment in the Late Assessment of Thrombolytic Efficacy (LATE) Study. *Journal of American College of Cardiology* Vol. 25, pp. 1063-1068.

Björklund, E., U. Stenestrand, J. Lindbäck, L. Svensson, L. Wallentin and B. Lindahl (2006). Pre-hospital thrombolysis delivered by paramedics is associated with reduced time delay and mortality in ambulance-transported real-life patients with ST-elevation myocardial infarction. *European Heart Journal*, Vol. 27,No. (10), pp. 1146-1152.

BNF (2011). *British National Formulary*, BMJ Group. London

Bonnefoy, E., P. G. Steg, F. Boutitie, P.-Y. Dubien, F. Lapostolle, J. Roncalli, F. Dissait, G. Vanzetto, A. Leizorowicz, G. Kirkorian and for the CAPTIM investigators (2009). Comparison of primary angioplasty and pre-hospital fibrinolysis in acute myocardial infarction (CAPTIM) trial: a 5-year follow-up. *European Heart Journal*, pp. ehp156.

European Society of Cardiology, (2008). Management of acute myocardial infarction in patients presenting with persistent ST-segment elevation: The Task Force on the management of ST-segment elevation acute myocardial infarction of the European Society of Cardiology. *Europen Heart Journal*, Vol. 29,No. (23), pp. 2909-2945.

Castle, N., C. Porter and B. Thompson (2007b). Acute myocardial infarction complicated by ventricular standstill terminated by thrombolysis and transcutaneous pacing. *Resuscitation*, Vol. 74,No. (3), pp. 559-562.

Castle, N. R., R. C. Owen and M. Hann (2007a). Is there still a place for emergency department thrombolysis following the introduction of the amended Joint Royal Colleges Ambulance Liaison Committee criteria for thrombolysis? *Emergency Medicine Journal*, Vol. 24,No. (12), pp. 843-845.

Chen, M., L. X. Jiang, Y. P. Chen, J. X. Xie, H. C. Pan, R. Peto, R. Collins and L. L.S (2005). Addition of clopidogrel to aspirin in 45 852 patients with acute myocardial infarction: randomised placebo-controlled trial. *The Lancet*, Vol. 366,No. (9497), pp. 1607-1621.

Cross, S. J., H. S. Lee, J. M. Rawles and K. Jennings (1991). Safety of thrombolysis in association with cardiopulmonary resuscitation. *British Medical Journal*, Vol. 303, pp. 1242.

Freimark D, M. S., Leor J, Boyto V et al. 2002; . (2002). Timing of aspirin administration as a determinant of survival of patients with acute myocardial infarction treated with thrombolysis. *American Journal of Cardiology*, Vol. 89, pp. 381-385.

Gore, J. M., C. B. Granger, M. L. Simoons, M. A. Sloan, W. D. Weaver, H. D. White, G. I. Barbash, F. Van de Werf, P. E. Aylward, E. J. Topol and R. M. Califf (1995). Stroke After Thrombolysis : Mortality and Functional Outcomes in the GUSTO-I Trial. *Circulation*, Vol. 92,No. (10), pp. 2811-2818.

EMIP Group. (1993). Prehospital thrombolytic therapy in patients with suspected acute myocardial infarction. *N Engl J Med* Vol. 329, pp. 383-390.

GUSTO (1993). An International Randomized Trial Comparing Four Thrombolytic Strategies for Acute Myocardial Infarction. *New England Journal of Medicine*, Vol. 329,No. (10), pp. 673-682.

Hoffmeister, H. M., M. Ruf, H. P. Wendel, W. Heller and L. Seipel (1998). Streptokinase-Induced Activation of the Kallikrein-Kinin System and of the Contact Phase in Patients with Acute Myocardial Infarction. *Journal of Cardiovascular Pharmacology*, Vol. 31,No. (5), pp. 764-772.

Horne, S., C. Weston, T. Quinn, A. Hicks, L. Walker, R. Chen and J. Birkhead (2009). The impact of pre-hospital thrombolytic treatment on re-infarction rates: analysis of the Myocardial Infarction National Audit Project (MINAP). *Heart*, Vol. 95,No. (7), pp. 559-563.

ISIS-2 (1988). Randomised Trial Of Intravenous Streptokinase, Oral Aspirin, Both, Or Neither Among 17 187 Cases Of Suspected Acute Myocardial Infarction: ISIS-2. *Lancet* Vol. 332,No. (8607), pp. 349.

Keeley, E. C., J. A. Boura and C. L. Grines (2006). Comparison of primary and facilitated percutaneous coronary interventions for ST-elevation myocardial infarction: quantitative review of randomised trials. *The Lancet*, Vol. 367,No. (9510), pp. 579-588.

Koren, G., A. T. Weiss, Y. Hasin, D. Appelbaum, S. Welber, Y. Rozenman, C. Lotan, M. Mosseri, D. Sapoznikov, M. H. Luria and M. S. Gotsman (1985). Prevention of Myocardial Damage in Acute Myocardial Ischemia by Early Treatment with Intravenous Streptokinase. *New England Journal of Medicine*, Vol. 313,No. (22), pp. 1384-1389.

Le May, M. R., R. F. Davies, R. Dionne, J. Maloney, J. Trickett, D. So, A. Ha, H. Sherrard, C. Glover, J.-F. Marquis, E. R. O'Brien, I. G. Stiell, P. Poirier and M. Labinaz (2006). Comparison of Early Mortality of Paramedic-Diagnosed ST-Segment Elevation Myocardial Infarction With Immediate Transport to a Designated Primary Percutaneous Coronary Intervention Center to That of Similar Patients Transported to the Nearest Hospital. *The American Journal of Cardiology*, Vol. 98,No. (10), pp. 1329-1333.

Lew, A., P. Laramee, B. Cercek, L. Rodriguez, P. Shah and W. Ganz (1985). The effects of the rate of intravenous infusion of streptokinase and the duration of symptoms on the time interval to reperfusion in patients with acute myocardial infarction. *Circulation*, Vol. 72,No. (5), pp. 1053-1058.

Liem, S.-S., B. L. van der Hoeven, P. V. Oemrawsingh, J. J. Bax, J. G. van der Bom, J. Bosch, E. P. Viergever, C. van Rees, I. Padmos, M. I. Sedney, H. J. van Exel, H. F. Verwey, D. E. Atsma, E. T. van der Velde, J. W. Jukema, E. E. van der Wall and M. J. Schalij (2007). MISSION!: Optimization of acute and chronic care for patients with acute myocardial infarction. *American Heart Journal*, Vol. 153,No. (1), pp. 14.e11-14.e11.

Mahaffey, K., C. Granger, C. Toth, H. White, A. Stebbins, G. Barbash, A. Vahanian, E. Topol and R. Califf (1997). Diabetic retinopathy should not be a contraindication to thrombolytic therapy for acute myocardial infarction: review of ocular hemorrhage incidence and location in the GUSTO-I trial. Global Utilization of Streptokinase and t-PA for Occluded Coronary Arteries. *J Am Coll Cardiol*, Vol. 30,No. (7), pp. 1606-1610.

Mannisi, J. A., H. F. Weisman, D. E. Bush, P. Dudeck and B. Healy (1987). Steroid administration after myocardial infarction promotes early infarct expansion. A study in the rat. *The Journal of Clinical Investigation*, Vol. 79,No. (5), pp. 1431-1439.

McLean, S., G. Egan, P. Connor and A. D. Flapan (2008). Collaborative decision-making between paramedics and CCU nurses based on 12-lead ECG telemetry expedites the delivery of thrombolysis in ST elevation myocardial infarction. *Emerg Med J*, Vol. 25,No. (6), pp. 370-374.

Mehta, R. H., C. K. Montoye, M. Gallogly, P. Baker, A. Blount, J. Faul, C. Roychoudhury, S. Borzak, S. Fox, M. Franklin, M. Freundl, E. Kline-Rogers, T. LaLonde, M. Orza, R. Parrish, M. Satwicz, M. J. Smith, P. Sobotka, S. Winston, A. A. Riba, K. A. Eagle and G. A. P. S. C. o. t. A. C. o. C. for the (2002). Improving Quality of Care for Acute Myocardial Infarction: The Guidelines Applied in Practice (GAP) Initiative. *JAMA*, Vol. 287,No. (10), pp. 1269-1276.

Morrison, L. J., P. R. Verbeek, A. C. McDonald, B. V. Sawadsky and D. J. Cook (2000). Mortality and Prehospital Thrombolysis for Acute Myocardial Infarction. *JAMA: The Journal of the American Medical Association*, Vol. 283,No. (20), pp. 2686-2692.

Morrow, D. A., E. M. Antman, K. A. A. Fox, H. D. White, R. Giugliano, S. A. Murphy, C. H. McCabe and E. Braunwald (2010). One-year outcomes after a strategy using enoxaparin vs. unfractionated heparin in patients undergoing fibrinolysis for ST-segment elevation myocardial infarction: 1-year results of the ExTRACT-TIMI 25 Trial. *European Heart Journal*, Vol. 31,No. (17), pp. 2097-2102.

Murphy, S. A., C. M. Gibson, D. A. Morrow, F. Van de Werf, I. B. Menown, S. G. Goodman, K. W. Mahaffey, M. Cohen, C. H. McCabe, E. M. Antman and E. Braunwald (2007). Efficacy and safety of the low-molecular weight heparin enoxaparin compared with unfractionated heparin across the acute coronary syndrome spectrum: a meta-analysis. *European Heart Journal*, Vol. 28,No. (17), pp. 2077-2086.

Neumar, R. W., Otto, C. W., Link, M. S., Kronick, S. L., Shuster, M., Callaway, C. W., Kudenchok, P. J., Ornato, J. P., McNally, B., Silvers, S. M., Passman, R. S., White, R. D., Hess, E. P., Tang, W., Davies, D., Sinz, E. & Morrison, L. J. (2010). Part 8: Adult Cardiovascular Life Support: 2010 American Heart Association Guidelines for Cardiopulmonary Resuscitation and Emergency Care. *Circulation*, Vol. Vol 122,No. (Supplement), pp. S729-S767.

O'Driscoll, B. R., Howard, L.S. & Davison, A.G. (2008). Guidelines for emergency oxygen use in adults: On behalf of the British Thoracic Society Emergency Oxygeng Guidelines Development Group. *Thorax*, Vol. 63,No. (Supplement VI), pp. VI 1-VI 73.

Opie, L. H. G., B. J. (2009). *Drugs for the heart.*, Saunders Elsevier. 978-4160-6158-8, Philadelphia

Rawles, J. (1994). Halving of mortality by domiciliary thrombolysis in the Grampian Reagion Early Anstreplase Trial (GREAT). *Journal of the American College of Cardiology*, Vol. 23, pp. 1-5.

Rawles, J. (2003). GREAT: 10 year survival of patients with suspected acute myocardial infarction in a randomised comparison of prehospital and hospital thrombolysis. *Heart*, Vol. 89,No. (5), pp. 563-564.

Rawles, J. M. (1997). Quantification of the Benefit of Earlier Thrombolytic Therapy: Five-Year Results of the Grampian Region Early Anistreplase Trial (GREAT). *Journal of the American College of Cardiology*, Vol. 30,No. (5), pp. 1181-1186.

Sabatine, M. S., C. P. Cannon, C. M. Gibson, J. L. López-Sendón, G. Montalescot, P. Theroux, B. S. Lewis, S. A. Murphy, C. H. McCabe and E. Braunwald (2005). Effect of Clopidogrel Pretreatment Before Percutaneous Coronary Intervention in Patients With ST-Elevation Myocardial Infarction Treated With Fibrinolytics. *JAMA: The Journal of the American Medical Association*, Vol. 294,No. (10), pp. 1224-1232.

Scirica, B. M., M. S. Sabatine, D. A. Morrow, C. M. Gibson, S. A. Murphy, S. D. Wiviott, R. P. Giugliano, C. H. McCabe, C. P. Cannon and E. Braunwald (2006). The Role of Clopidogrel in Early and Sustained Arterial Patency After Fibrinolysis for ST-Segment Elevation Myocardial Infarction: The ECG CLARITY-TIMI 28 Study. *Journal of American College of Cardiology*, Vol. 48,No. (1), pp. 37-42.

Tatu-Chiţoiu, G., C. Teodorescu, M. Dan, M. Guran, P. Căpraru, O. Istrăţescu, A. Tatu-Chiţoiu, A. Bumbu, V. Chioncel, S. Arvanitopol and M. Dorobanţu (2004). Streptokinase-induced hypotension has no detrimental effect on patients with thrombolytic treatment for acute myocardial infarction. A substudy of the Romanian Study for Accelerated Streptokinase in Acute Myocardial   Infarction (ASK-ROMANIA). *Romanian Journal of Internal Medicine*, Vol. 42,No. (3), pp. 557-573.

van 't Hof, A. W. J., S. Rasoul, H. van de Wetering, N. Ernst, H. Suryapranata, J. C. A. Hoorntje, J.-H. E. Dambrink, M. Gosselink, F. Zijlstra, J. P. Ottervanger and M.-J. de Boer (2006). Feasibility and benefit of prehospital diagnosis, triage, and therapy by paramedics only in patients who are candidates for primary angioplasty for acute myocardial infarction. *American Heart Journal*, Vol. 151,No. (6), pp. 1255.e1251-1255.e1255.

Van de Werf, F., J. Bax, A. Betriu, C. Blomstrom-Lundqvist, F. Crea, V. Falk, G. Filippatos, K. Fox, K. Huber, A. Kastrati, A. Rosengren, P. G. Steg, M. Tubaro, F. Verheugt, F. Weidinger, M. Weis, E. C. f. P. Guidelines, A. Vahanian, J. Camm, R. De Caterina, V. Dean, K. Dickstein, C. Funck-Brentano, I. Hellemans, S. D. Kristensen, K. McGregor, U. Sechtem, S. Silber, M. Tendera, P. Widimsky, J. L. Zamorano, D. Reviewers, F. V. Aguirre, N. Al-Attar, E. Alegria, F. Andreotti, W. Benzer, O. Breithardt, N. Danchin, C. D. Mario, D. Dudek, D. Gulba, S. Halvorsen, P. Kaufmann, R. Kornowski, G. Y. H. Lip and F. Rutten (2008). Management of acute myocardial infarction in patients presenting with persistent ST-segment elevation. *European Heart Journal*, Vol. 29,No. (23), pp. 2909-2945.

Van de Werf, P., A. Ross, P. Armstrong and C. Granger (2006). Primary versus tenecteplase-facilitated percutaneous coronary intervention in patients with ST-segment elevation acute myocardial infarction (ASSENT-4 PCI): randomised trial. *The Lancet*, Vol. 367,No. (9510), pp. 569-578.

Wallentin, L., P. Goldstein, P. W. Armstrong, C. B. Granger, A. A. J. Adgey, H. R. Arntz, K. Bogaerts, T. Danays, B. Lindahl, M. Mäkijärvi, F. Verheugt and F. Van de Werf (2003). Efficacy and Safety of Tenecteplase in Combination With the Low-Molecular-Weight Heparin Enoxaparin or Unfractionated Heparin in the Prehospital Setting. *Circulation*, Vol. 108,No. (2), pp. 135-142.

Weaver, W. D., Simes R.J., Betriu, A., Grines, C.L., Zijistra, F., Garcia, E., Grinfield, L., Gibbons, E.E., DeWood, M.A., Ribichini, F. (1997). Comparison of primary coronary angioplasty and intravenous thrombolytic therapy for acute myocardial infarction: a quantitative review. *Journal of American Medical Association* Vol. 278,No. (23), pp. 2093-2098.

Welsh, R. C., A. Travers, M. Senaratne, R. Williams and P. W. Armstrong (2006). Feasibility and applicability of paramedic-based prehospital fibrinolysis in a large North American center. *American Heart Journal*, Vol. 152,No. (6), pp. 1007.

Westerhout, C. M., E. Bonnefoy, R. C. Welsh, P. G. Steg, F. Boutitie and P. W. Armstrong (2011). The influence of time from symptom onset and reperfusion strategy on 1-year survival in ST-elevation myocardial infarction: A pooled analysis of an early fibrinolytic strategy versus primary percutaneous coronary intervention from CAPTIM and WEST. *American Heart Journal*, Vol. 161,No. (2), pp. 283-290.

Yusuf, S., F. Zhao, S. R. Mehta, S. Chrolavicius, G. Tognoni and K. K. Fox (2001). Effects of Clopidogrel in Addition to Aspirin in Patients with Acute Coronary Syndromes without ST-Segment Elevation. *New England Journal of Medicine*, Vol. 345,No. (7), pp. 494-502.

8

Platelet Activation in Ischemic Heart Disease: Role of Modulators and New Therapies

Mahdi Garelnabi[1], Javier E. Horta[1] and Emir Veledar[2]
[1]Department of Clinical Laboratory and Nutritional Sciences
University of Massachusetts Lowell, Lowell, MA
[2]Emory University School of Medicine Atlanta, GA
USA

1. Introduction

Ischemic heart disease (IHD) remains the major cause of morbidity and mortality in developed countries, and has joined infectious diseases in developing countries as a leading cause of death (WHO 2008). Decades of research have shown conclusively that a number of determinants operating from early childhood onwards, most of them associated with lifestyle, are responsible for IHD.

IHD results when the oxygen demand of the myocardium cannot be met due to an inadequate blood supply. The most common cause of myocardial ischemia is atherosclerosis of epicardial coronary arteries. The major risk factors for atherosclerosis, and therefore IHD, are dyslipidemia (i.e., elevated low-density lipoprotein (LDL) and/or low high-density lipoprotein (HDL)), diabetes mellitus, hypertension, cigarette smoking, poor dietary habits, and lack of physical activity. These risk factors, particularly when more than one co-exists, can progressively damage the vascular endothelium, causing dysregulation of its anti-inflammatory and anti-thrombotic functions. The associated proliferation of underlying fibroblasts and vascular myocytes, together with the accumulation of extracellular matrix and lipids, result in the formation of what are known as atherosclerotic plaques that lead to a reduction in the luminal diameter. Some of the risk factors for atherosclerosis facilitate the development of atherosclerotic plaques, while others sustain or accelerate their formation, producing the clinical manifestations of IHD (Parthasarathy 2008, Garelnabi 2010).

By reducing the lumen of blood vessels, atherosclerosis causes an absolute decrease in myocardial perfusion in the basal state and hinders the required increase in perfusion when the demand for flow is augmented. As this process progressively worsens, the shear stress associated with blood flow through the reduced arterial lumen can cause plaques to erode or rupture, exposing the intimal layer to the luminal contents and thereby promoting frank thrombosis. Platelet activation, mobilization, and recruitment are central to this process. Luminal thrombi can trap red blood cells and acutely reduce coronary blood flow, producing a sudden myocardial ischemic event referred to as an acute coronary syndrome (ACS) that becomes manifest as either unstable angina or myocardial infarction (MI) if there is complete occlusion without prompt reperfusion. MI may also occur with embolization of platelet aggregates and/or atherosclerotic debris from a ruptured plaque.

Coronary blood flow can also be limited by vascular spasm, as well as by congenital abnormalities, such as anomalous origin of the left anterior descending coronary artery from the pulmonary artery, which may cause myocardial ischemia and infarction in infancy, but is very rare in adults.

Patients with IHD can be grouped into two broad categories: those having chronic coronary artery disease (CAD), who most commonly present with stable angina, and those who present with ACSs (i.e., unstable angina and MI). Chronic CAD is most commonly caused by slowly progressive coronary artery atherosclerosis, whereby a narrowing of the lumen of the coronary arteries limits their ability to adequately increase perfusion in response to an increase in demand for oxygen (e.g., during exertion). As the disease progresses in severity, perfusion of the myocardium can become compromised even at rest. ACSs, on the other hand, are the result of acute vasoocclusive events secondary to thrombosis at sites of erosion or rupture of atherosclerotic lesions.

2. Role of platelets in the etiology and pathophysiology of IHD

2.1 Structure of platelets

Blood platelets play an essential role in hemostasis, thrombosis, and coagulation of blood. They are engaged in a complex repertoire of biochemical and molecular activities designed to prevent hemorrhage.

On Wright-Giemsa-stained blood smears, platelets appear as small, anucleate, ovoid or round cells with a pale grayish blue cytoplasm that contains homogeneously distributed purple-red granules. After platelet spreading or aggregation, these dispersed granules become concentrated in the middle of the cell.

When platelet morphology is considered under functional subdivisions rather than purely anatomic terms, there are three major structural zones of the platelet, each related to specific aspect of platelet function. The peripheral zone is involved primarily in adhesion, the solgel zone in contraction, and the organelle zone in secretion.

The volumes of circulating platelets from a single individual are heterogeneous and exhibit a log normal size distribution. Circulating platelets have a volume of 7.06 ± 4.85 μm^3 (femtoliters), a diameter of 3.6 ± 0.7 μm (Mean $\pm$ SD), and a thickness of 0.9 ± 0.3 μm (Paulus et al. 1979, Frojmovic et al. 1976). Platelet size varies from one individual to another, although abnormally small or large platelets are present only in certain disease states. By scanning electron microscopy, circulating blood platelets appear as flat discs, with smooth contours and rare spiny filopodia, with random openings of a channel system, which invaginates throughout the platelet and is the conduit by which granule contents exocytose after stimulation. Although the platelet is anucleate, transmission electron microscopy reveals a cytoplasm packed with a number of different organelles essential to maintenance of normal hemostasis. Platelets contain four distinct populations of granules: α-granules, dense bodies, lysosomes, and microperoxisomes. α-granules and dense bodies are distinguished morphologically from one another by their electron density as revealed by electron microscopy.

Phospholipids constitute 80% of the total lipid content of platelets, although smaller amounts of neutral lipids and glycolipids are also present. Evidence suggests that these phospholipids move to the outer membrane leaflet after platelet activation, thereby functioning to promote clot formation. Platelet membrane glycoproteins mediate a wide number of adhesive cellular interactions. These glycoproteins function as receptors that can receive signals from outside the platelet, facilitating cell-cell interactions; binding of specific ligands to these receptors results in distinct platelet responses to the external environment. Several other proteins are unique to the platelet, including platelet factor 4 (PF4), low-affinity PF4, β-thromboglobulin (β-TG), and the calcium-binding proteins thrombospondin, calmodulin, and platelet-derived growth factor (PDGF) (Stenberg et al. 1984).

2.2 Function and biochemistry of platelets

In terms of dry weight, platelets are composed of approximately 60% protein, 15% lipid, and 8% carbohydrate. Platelet minerals include magnesium, calcium, potassium, and zinc. Platelets contain substantial amounts of vitamin B_{12}, folic acid, and ascorbic acid (Weiss et al. 1968). The concentration of sodium and potassium within the platelet are 39 and 138 mEq, respectively, a gradient against plasma that is maintained by active ion pumping, which derives energy from membrane adenosine triphosphatase of the Ouabain-sensitive, Na^+/K^+-dependent type. Potassium apparently is distributed in two discrete metabolic compartments (Cooley and Cohen 1967).

Non-stimulated platelets maintain a low cytoplasmic Ca^{2+} concentration, by limiting Ca^{2+} transport from plasma and promoting active efflux of this ion from the cell. Two pools of calcium are present in platelets: a rapidly-turning over cytosolic pool that is regulated by sodium-calcium antiporter in the plasma membrane, and a more slowly-exchanging pool that is regulated by a calcium-magnesium-ATPase and is sequestered in a dense tubular system. Platelets are therefore able to transport calcium from the cytosol by moving it against a gradient into the extracellular space or by sequestration in the dense tubular system (Brass 1984, Enouf et al. 1987).

There are several similarities between the energy metabolism of platelets and that of skeletal muscle. Both involve active glycolysis and the synthesis and use of large amounts of glycogen, and in both, the major mediator of intracellular energy use is ATP. Platelets, like muscle cells, are metabolically adapted to expend large amounts of energy rapidly during aggregation, the release reaction, and clot retraction (Karpatkin et al. 1970).

The presence of platelets in the hemostatic plugs that form to prevent bleeding suggests that platelets have a physiological role in hemostasis. Their presence in thrombi and emboli, however, suggests that they may have a pathological role as well. Platelets display certain properties that may be relevant to hemostasis and thrombosis. They have the capacity to adhere to foreign surfaces, they can be induced to aggregate, and they can synthesize or release a number of substances.

Platelet adhesion

The only structures with which platelets normally interact are red cells, white cells, and the endothelial lining of blood vessel walls. All other surfaces are thus foreign to them, but platelets have the ability to adhere to such surfaces. Platelets adhere to subendothelial structures that are exposed when the normal endothelial lining of the blood vessel wall is injured, which causes the deposition of a monolayer of platelets on the surface of the injured vessel. This is followed by the release of pro-coagulation substances, leading to platelet aggregation and formation of a fibrin clot over the adhered layer that results in thrombus formation (Heptinstall and Hanley 1985).

Platelet aggregation

Platelets circulate as disc-shaped cells, but when they come in contact with exposed subendothelium, agonists that activate platelets are exposed, generated, or released. These agonists include collagen, which is present in subendothelium; thrombin, which is generated on the surface of activated platelets and elsewhere; ADP, which is released from damaged red blood cells and secreted from activated platelet-dense granules; circulating epinephrine; and arachidonic acid, which is released from lipid stores in platelets and metabolized to the potent agonist thromboxane A_2 (TXA_2). These agonists generally cause platelets to change shape such that they form long pseudopodia, followed by platelet aggregation. Aggregation requires activation of platelet integrin adhesion receptor GP IIb/IIIa so that it can bind fibrinogen or von Willebrand factor (vWF) and link adjacent platelets together in an aggregate. Platelet agonists induce signal transduction events in platelets that cause the above events, although the signal transduction pathways are not completely understood (Leslie et al. 1999).

Platelet release reaction

Platelets store ATP, ADP, Ca^{2+}, and serotonin in dense granules as well as adhesive proteins such as platelet factor 4, β-thromboglobulin, platelet-derived growth factor (PDGF), fibrinogen, fibronectin, thrombospondin, and vWF in α-granules (Siess 1989). Upon activation by agonists, platelets undergo a release reaction, thereby secreting their granular contents. The release reaction is associated with the production of TXA_2, and the extent of the secretion depends on the strength of the agonist. Weak agonists (e.g., ADP and epinephrine) require both cyclooxygenase activity and primary aggregation to induce secretion that is observed at low Ca^{2+} concentrations (Smith et al. 1973, Banga et al. 1986). Agonists of intermediate strength (e.g., platelet activating factor, PAF) can induce secretion in the absence of formation of arachidonic acid metabolism and without primary aggregation. Interestingly, when collagen is added at low concentrations to platelet suspensions, secretion of ATP occurs before the onset of shape change. This secretion is not inhibited by cyclooxygenase blockers, but is sensitive to the extracellular Ca^{2+} concentration and is a direct consequence of platelet binding to collagen (Siess et al. 1983, Malmgren 1986).

Platelet activation

Some signaling pathways involved in various platelet activation events are reasonably well understood, whereas others are not. Many, but not all platelet agonists activate platelets by occupying seven transmembrane-spanning, G protein-coupled receptors. Activation of these receptors generally results in activation of phospholipase Cβ (PLC). PLC hydrolyzes phosphatidyl-inositol-4,5-bisphosphate (PIP_2), generating inositol-1,4,5-triphosphate (IP_3) and diacylglycerol (DAG). Both IP_3 and DAG appear to play important roles in pathways leading to various aspects of platelet activation. IP_3 is believed to interact with specific receptors to induce intracellular Ca^{2+} release from the dense tubular system, an intracellular

Ca^{2+} storage organelle analogous to the sarcoplasmic reticulum in skeletal muscle. However, the exact mechanism by which this response contributes to platelet aggregation is not entirely clear because IP_3-induced platelet aggregation is also dependent on thromboxane A_2 (TXA_2) production and ADP release (Knezevic et al. 1992). DAG interacts directly with protein kinase C (PKC) and appears to play a crucial role in the pathways of some agonists, leading to the activation of GP IIb/IIIa and fibrinogen binding. Specific inhibitors of PKC block fibrinogen binding and platelet aggregation induced by some agonists. Drivers for platelet activation include the signaling events that occur downstream of receptors for collagen (GP VI and GP Ibα), thrombin (PAR1 and PAR4), adenosine diphosphate (ADP; P2Y1 and P2Y12), and thromboxane A2 (TXA_2; TP) (Brass 2010).

Platelets are activated and stimulated to synthesize or release a number of substances, namely thrombin, arachidonic acid, PAF, and epinephrine which are of functional importance. When platelet ADP is released from platelet-dense granules during platelet activation by numerous agonists, secreted ADP potentiates the activating effects of other agonists (Hourani and Cusack 1991). ADP causes shape change, granular secretion, and aggregation. However, unlike strong agonists such as thrombin and collagen, ADP induces secretion usually only in conjunction with platelet aggregation. Strong agonists generally stimulate phosphoinositide hydrolysis, increase cytosolic free Ca^{2+}, and induce TXA_2 formation.

Platelet receptors and MicroRNA signaling

Platelet receptors are known to interact with external stimuli in the main blood stream leading to the regulation of platelet activation. Platelet adhesion receptors are the key initiators of platelet activation at sites of vascular injury, where platelets become exposed to adhesive proteins in the matrix, or on endothelial cells. Despite significant differences in their functions and signaling pathways, several major platelet adhesion receptors share many similarities in their signal transduction mechanisms (Li et al. 2010). The most studied platelet receptor is platelet integrin GP IIb/IIIa, which is reported to play an essential role in thrombus formation through interactions with adhesive ligands and has emerged as a primary target for the development of anti-thrombotic agents (Hagemeyer and Peter 2010). Successful blockade of this ligand binding has validated GP IIb/IIIa as a therapeutic target in cardiovascular medicine.

MicroRNAs (MiRs) molecules are a novel class of endogenous, small, noncoding RNAs that regulate gene expression via degradation, translational inhibition, or translational activation of their target messenger RNAs (Pan et al. 2010, O'Sullivan et al., 2011). Bioinformatics analysis predicts that each MiR can regulate hundreds of targets, suggesting that they play an essential role in almost every physiological and pathological pathway. Functionally, an individual MiR is important as a transcription factor because it is able to regulate the expression of its multiple target genes. MiRs are short (~20 nucleotides long), single-stranded RNAs initially transcribed by either RNA polymerase II or RNA polymerase III, as a long primary MiR transcript (pre-MiR). It is then cleaved in the nucleus by the microprocessor complex, Drosha-DGCR8, resulting in a precursor hairpin (pre-miRNA) ranging in length from 60 to 110 nucleotides. The pre-MiRNA is exported from the nucleus to the cytoplasm by exportin 5-Ran-GTP. In the cytoplasm, Dicer, a member of the RNase III family, in complex with TRBP, cleaves the pre-MiR hairpin to a 22 base pair MiR duplex.

The mature MiR is incorporated with argonaute (Ago2) proteins into the RNA-induced silencing complex (RISC), where MiR guides the complex to partial complementary binding sites located in the 3′ untranslated region (UTR) of target mRNAs to suppress gene expression. MiRs are able to directly regulate at least 30% of genes in a cell. In addition, other genes may also be regulated indirectly by MiRs. Therefore, MiRs are pivotal regulators in normal development, physiology, and pathology. Recent studies have identified a number of MiRs highly expressed in the vasculature and their expression is dysregulated in diseased vessels (Jamaluddin et al. 2011, Haver et al. 2010, Bonauer et al. 2010, Wierda et al. 2010, Urbich et al. 2008, Fang et al. 2010, Leeper et al. 2011). MiRs are also found to be critical modulators of cell differentiation, contraction, migration, proliferation, and apoptosis. Accordingly, MiRs have emerged as therapeutic targets in disease.

Platelets are also reported to have microRNA population that may regulate its activity. It is well known that platelets have mRNA and mRNA splicing machinery, and translate mRNA into proteins relevant to hemostasis and inflammation (Edelstein and Bray 2011). In silicon analysis work from Edelstein and Bray indicates that each platelet MiR targets an average of 307 distinct mRNAs, concluding in their review that platelet MiRs have ample opportunity to regulate platelet function.

2.3 Role of inflammation and oxidative stress in platelet activation

Involvement of inflammation in cardiovascular disease is well defined. Circulating platelets are affected by this metabolic disruption and by inflammatory mediators synthesized and/or released on contact with inflammatory signals. Platelets are known to play a major role in this process and have been identified as targets and players in inflammation-induced cardiovascular disease (Weksler 1983, Nurden 2011). It has been explicitly established that free radicals can cause metabolic disturbances and cell injury in a variety of ways, including lipid peroxidation, hydroxyl radical-induced modification of proteins and nucleic acids, changes in enzyme activity, and carbohydrate damage. Oxidative modification of lipids can be induced in vitro by a wide array of pro-oxidant agents and occurs in vivo during atherosclerosis and several other disease conditions (Parthasarathy et al. 2008). Alterations in the superoxide and glutathione oxidation-reduction system may lead to depleted antioxidant capacity and may result in oxidative stress. Previous studies have suggested that platelets and vascular endothelial cells could be the central target as well as the origin of oxygen free radicals or its metabolites (Dousset et al. 1983). Measuring the end products of lipid peroxidation is one of the most widely accepted assays for oxidative damage. These aldehydic secondary products of lipid peroxidation are generally accepted markers of oxidative stress.

Several studies suggest that the basal release of NO by the endothelium contributes to regulation of the vascular tone (Antoniades et al. 2008), blood flow, and blood pressure. NO inhibits platelet aggregation and adhesion to vascular endothelium. In addition, NO inhibits leukocyte adhesion to endothelium (Petidis et al. 2008). Alteration of cellular calcium homeostasis is also a critical event in ischemic heart injury. NO released by endothelium or synthesized by platelets participates in the regulation of Ca^{2+} signaling. Elevation of cGMP as a result of the activation of guanylate cyclase by NO stimulates a number of mechanisms that actively decrease calcium levels within the cell (Joseph et al. 1996). Although the NO-cGMP signaling system has been immensely investigated, sparse data is available pertaining to the role of platelet NO activity in coronary artery (CAD). We and others have studied the NO-cGMP system in patients with CAD, particularly the role of oxidative stress and NO-mediated platelet response in IHD (Garelnabi et al. 2010, Ikeda et al. 2000, Garelnabi et al. 2011). These studies have clearly indicated that lipid peroxidation is augmented in patients with ischemic heart disease. The increased oxidative stress seen in these patients was accompanied by platelet activation and impaired antioxidant enzymes activity. On the other hand, platelet aggregation, NO, cGMP, NO synthase activity, plasma NO, and ionized Ca^{2+} was profoundly increased in CAD. The increases in NO-cGMP components may have resulted as a compensatory response to ameliorate platelet activity and increased Ca^{2+} levels in CAD patients. Another interesting modulator of platelet activity is the recent description of platelet-derived microparticles (PMP) which are known as a heterogeneous population of vesicles (<1 mm) generated from the plasma membrane upon platelet activation by various stimuli. These PMPs have been shown to not only stimulate the response of platelets, but have also been reported to mediate the intercellular transfer of bioactive molecules such as lipids, surface receptors, and even enzymes (Siljander 2010).

3. Classes and mechanism of action of antiplatelet drugs

The main goals of pharmacological intervention in patients with IHD are to reduce the occurrence of anginal attacks by minimizing the rise in blood pressure and heart rate associated with physical activity so that patients can go about their daily activities without ischemic episodes. Given the prominent role that thrombosis plays in IHD, antiplatelet therapy is one of the most important modalities used in its treatment.

Antithrombotic drugs used for prevention and treatment of thrombosis include: (1) antiplatelet drugs, (2) anticoagulants, and (3) fibrinolytic agents. Given the predominance of platelets in arterial thrombi, which are the major source of IHD, the treatment and inhibition of arterial thrombosis focus mainly on antiplatelet agents, although anticoagulants and fibrinolytic drugs are often included in the acute setting.

Under normal conditions, the actions of vascular endothelial cells maintain platelets in the bloodstream in an inactive state, largely by their production of nitric oxide (NO) and prostacyclin, but also by their surface expression of adenosine diphosphatase (ADPase), which breaks down ADP released via degranulation of activated platelets. With the occurrence of injury to the vascular endothelium, production of these substances is compromised and certain components of the subendothelial matrix are exposed (e.g., collagen, von Willebrand factor (vWF), and fibronectin) to which platelets adhere via receptors constitutively expressed on their surface (e.g., GP IIb/IIIa). As discussed above, adhered platelets undergo a morphological change and then release the contents of their dense granules (e.g., ADP) and synthesize and release thromboxane A_2 (TXA_2), both of which serve to recruit and activate surrounding circulating platelets to the site of vascular injury.

Disruption of the vascular wall also exposes underlying cells and matrix that express pro-thrombotic factors to the circulation, which triggers the coagulation cascade. Activated platelets enhance coagulation by binding clotting factors and supporting the assembly of activation complexes that increase thrombin generation, which in addition to converting fibrinogen to fibrin, also acts as a potent platelet agonist and recruits more platelets to the site of vascular injury.

The most abundant receptor on the surface of platelets is GP IIb/IIIa, which undergoes a conformational change upon platelet activation that allows it to bind fibrinogen. Divalent fibrinogen molecules link adjacent platelets together to form aggregates, which are meshed together via fibrin strands generated via the action of thrombin to form a lattice composed of platelets plus fibrin. Antiplatelet drugs target various steps in this process. The most commonly used drugs include cyclooxygenase inhibitors, among which aspirin is the most common, thienopyridines and functionally related drugs, phosphodiesterase inhibitors, adenosine reuptake inhibitors, and GP IIb/IIIa antagonists, all of which are discussed below.

3.1 Cyclooxygenase inhibitors

The cyclooxygenases (COXs) are a family of isoenzymes responsible for the biosynthesis of various important and potent pro-inflammatory and pro-thrombotic mediators called eicosanoids, which include prostaglandins, leukotrienes, and thromboxanes. Non-steroidal anti-inflammatory drugs (NSAIDs), like aspirin and ibuprofen, exert their effects through inhibition of COX, and as such they relieve the symptoms of inflammation (e.g., pain, swelling).

COX converts arachidonic acid (AA, an ω-6 polyunsaturated fatty acid (PUFA)) to prostaglandin H_2 (PGH_2), the parent of the eicosanoids, which can then be converted to the other compounds via further enzymatic action that involves radical chemistry and the consumption of molecular oxygen. To date, three distinct COX isoenzymes have been identified: COX-1, COX-2, and COX-3. COX-1 and COX-3 are products of alternative splicing of the same gene, so COX-3 is referred to by some as COX-1b or COX-1 variant (COX-1v). Different tissues express varying levels of the different COXs, and although the isoenzymes basically catalyze the same transformations, selective inhibition can produce a different side-effect profile. COX-1 is nearly ubiquitous among mammalian cells, but COX-2 is undetectable in most normal tissues and is inducible in macrophages upon their activation, as well in endothelial cells at sites of inflammation, where it serves to produce prostacyclin, a potent vasodilator and inhibitor of platelet aggregation. COX-2 is also upregulated in various types of cancers, so it is believed to play a role in oncogenesis.

Both COX-1 and -2 also oxygenate two other essential fatty acids – dihomo-γ-linolenic acid (DGLA, ω-6) and eicosapentaenoic acid (EPA, ω-3) – to give eicosanoids with less potent pro-inflammatory properties than those derived from AA. Both DGLA and EPA competitively inhibit oxidation of AA by the COXs, which is believed to be the major mechanism by which dietary sources of DGLA and EPA (e.g., fish oil) can reduce inflammation.

The traditional COX inhibitors are not selective for any particular COX, resulting in widespread inhibition of eicosanoid synthesis that ultimately reduces inflammation, as well as providing antipyretic, antithrombotic, and analgesic effects. However, inhibition of the synthesis of gastroprotective prostaglandins can cause gastric irritation and increases the risk of development of peptic ulcer disease.

The development of selective COX-2 inhibitors was originally aimed at blocking the production of pro-inflammatory prostaglandins while minimizing any effects on platelet and gastric function. Selective inhibition of COX-2 has been accomplished with the "coxibs", which differ in their selectivity for COX-2 relative to COX-1 by selectively binding to a hydrophobic side-pocket on the COX-2 enzyme where a valine takes the place of what is an isoleucine on COX-1, allowing access to an otherwise sterically hindered site that causes inhibition of the enzyme's function. Since COX-2 is largely expressed selectively in inflamed tissue, there is much less gastric irritation and risk of peptic ulceration associated with COX-2 inhibitors. However, the selectivity of COX-2 causes an imbalance between thromboxane and prostacyclin, resulting in an increased risk of thrombosis, MI, and stroke. Thus, by blocking prostacyclin synthesis without concomitant inhibition of thromboxane A_2 (TXA_2) production, highly selective inhibitors of COX-2 increase the risk of cardiovascular events. These effects seemed most notable with rofecoxib (Vioxx®) and valdecoxib (Bextra®), which were removed from the market in 2004 and 2005, respectively. Other COX-2 selective NSAIDs, such as celecoxib (Celebrex®), and etoricoxib (Arcoxia®), are still on the market as they continue to be investigated for these adverse effects. Even with short-term use, COX-2 inhibitors have been found to increase the risk of atherothrombosis, most notably manifested as a 2-to-5-fold increased risk of myocardial infarction. Furthermore, high-dose regimens of some traditional NSAIDs such as diclofenac and ibuprofen are associated with a similar increase in risk of vascular events. Thus, although NSAIDs, particularly COX-2 inhibitors, have demonstrated benefits, the risks associated with their use should be seriously considered when prescribing them to a patient having risk factors and/or a personal or family history of IHD.

3.1.1 Aspirin

Aspirin (acetylsalicylic acid, ASA), is the oldest and most widely used antiplatelet drug due to its low cost, wide availability, and proven effectiveness. It is a salicylate drug whose mechanism of action serves as the model of most antiplatelet therapeutic strategies.

Mechanism of action

Aspirin, a non-selective COX inhibitor, is one of the most commonly used drugs in IHD that can reduce the development of thrombosis associated with the rupture of atheromatous plaques. Aspirin interferes with the activation of platelets by irreversibly inhibiting COX, thereby interfering with the biosynthetic pathway of thromboxanes. Unlike other NSAIDs, whose antiplatelet action is transient (i.e., in the order of hours), aspirin irreversibly acetylates COX-1 in platelets, thereby inhibiting the biosynthesis of thromboxane A_2 (TXA_2) and in that manner producing a long-lived antithrombotic effect (i.e., days, until new platelets are produced by the bone marrow). At higher doses (e.g., 1 g/d), however, aspirin also inhibits COX-2, which can ultimately produce a prothrombotic effect by inhibiting the synthesis of prostacyclin in endothelial cells.

Indications, dosage, and side effects

Aspirin is widely used for the primary prevention of ischemic events in patients at risk, as well as secondary prevention of cardiovascular events in patients with IHD and cerebrovascular and peripheral vascular disease. Aspirin is usually administered once a day at a dose between 75-325 mg, with 75-100 mg being recommended for most indications. When fast platelet inhibition is needed, a dose of at least 160 mg should be given orally. Higher doses of aspirin have not been shown to be more effective than lower doses, and in fact, reduced efficacy has been reported with higher doses. As discussed above, very high doses of aspirin (i.e., 1 g/d) can have a paradoxical prothrombotic effect due to the inhibition of COX-2.

Long-term daily oral enteric-coated aspirin has been demonstrated to reduce (1) the incidence of anginal episodes in patients with chronic stable angina, as well as in survivors of unstable angina and myocardial infarction (MI), and (2) the risk of recurrent infarction, stroke, or cardiovascular mortality by 25% following an MI compared with placebo. It has also been established that low doses of aspirin may be given immediately after an MI to reduce the risk of another MI or of the death of the myocardium.

Aspirin is equally effective in men and women, although in men it mainly reduces the risk of MI, while in women it lowers the risk of stroke. Although aspirin also raises the risk of hemorrhagic stroke and other major bleeds, these events are rare, and are by far outweighed by aspirin's positive effects.

The most common side effects of aspirin use are gastrointestinal, ranging from simple stomach upset, to erosive gastritis, to peptic ulcers with bleeding and perforation, all of which are dose-dependent. For these reasons, aspirin should never be administered to individuals with a history of gastrointestinal bleeding or severe stomach upset. Although the use of enteric-coated or buffered aspirin may relieve some of these symptoms, they do not eliminate the risk of gastrointestinal complications due to the inhibition of gastroprotective prostaglandins as part of the actions of aspirin. The overall risk of major bleeding with aspirin is low, however, estimated at 1-3% per year, but is increased when aspirin is given in conjunction with anticoagulants (e.g., warfarin). In these situations, a lower dose of aspirin should be given (e.g., 75-100 mg/d). In patients with a documented history of peptic ulcer disease caused by Helicobacter pylori infection, treatment of the infection and administration of a proton pump inhibitor (PPI) may reduce the risk of aspirin-induced gastrointestinal bleeding. Aspirin should also never be given to individuals with a history of allergic responses to salicylates, particularly those associated with bronchospasm.

3.2 Thienopyridines

A second class of antiplatelet drugs commonly used in IHD is the thienopyridines. These structurally related drugs have similar benefits as aspirin in patients with stable chronic IHD and may be used instead of aspirin when aspirin is contraindicated. The thienopyridines include clopidogrel (Plavix®), ticlopidine (Ticlid®), and prasugrel (Effient®). A structurally unrelated but functionally similar drug is ticagrelor (Brilinta®).

Mechanism of action

The thienopyridines are prodrugs that must first be metabolized by the hepatic cytochrome P450 enzyme system before they can exert any biological activity, so their onset of action can be delayed for several days. They interfere with the aggregation of platelets by competitively and irreversibly inhibiting the adenosine diphosphate (ADP) chemoreceptor P2Y12 on the surface of platelets, which is crucial for the conformational change that activates GP IIb/IIIa and ultimately leads to platelet aggregation and cross-linking by fibrin.

3.2.1 Clopidogrel (Plavix®)

Clopidogrel is an oral thienopyridine marketed under the trade name Plavix by Bristol-Myers Squibb and Sanofi-Aventis as 75 mg oral tablets.

Indications, dosage, and side effects

Clopidogrel is indicated for the prevention of vascular ischemic events in patients with symptomatic atherosclerosis, acute coronary syndromes, and MI. When compared with aspirin in patients with recent ischemic stroke, MI, or peripheral arterial disease, clopidogrel further reduced the risk of cardiovascular death, MI, and stroke by nearly 10%. Thus, although clopidogrel is actually more effective than aspirin in reducing morbidity and mortality of IHD, it is also considerably more expensive and not as readily available. It is also used, together with aspirin, for the prevention of thrombotic events after placement of intracoronary stents, or as an alternative to aspirin in patients who have a contraindication for aspirin.

Combination therapy consisting of aspirin and clopidogrel has been shown to reduce morbidity and mortality in patients with angina and it also reduces the risk of thrombosis in patients who have undergone coronary artery stenting (the risk of gastrointestinal bleeding in these patients can be reduced by also prescribing a PPI while on this combination therapy). The combination therapy of clopidogrel and aspirin capitalizes on the capacity of these drugs to inhibit complementary pathways of platelet activation and is associated with a highly statistically significant 20% relative risk reduction when comparing each drug alone.

In patients with a history of acute coronary syndrome, it is standard medical practice to administer aspirin indefinitely, and it is recommended that combination therapy with clopidogrel be given for 1-3 months after the implantation of a bare metal stent. With the use of drug-eluting stents, which deliver antiproliferative drugs locally (e.g., rapamycin or paclitaxel), combination therapy should continue for at least one year because these drugs are associated with delayed endothelial healing that prolongs the window during which there is an increased risk for thrombosis around the area where the stent was placed. Although aspirin and clopidogrel may help prevent coronary thrombosis associated with stenting, there is no evidence that these drugs reduce the occurrence of re-stenosis. However, the use of drug-eluting stents can reduce re-stenosis to near zero within the stent itself and less than 10% at its edges.

There is little evidence of additional benefit of adding clopidogrel to the routine regimen of aspirin in patients with chronic stable IHD that have not undergone stenting. However, "aspirin resistance" has been noted in up to 10% of patients, more frequently in patients treated with lower doses of aspirin. In these cases, the use of higher doses of aspirin and/or combination therapy with clopidogrel should be considered. Although the routine management of patients with IHD is medical, many patients show greater improvement after undergoing interventional coronary revascularization. These invasive procedures should not take the place of the required ongoing modification of risk factors and medical therapy but rather should be performed in combination with them.

Combination therapy of aspirin and clopidogrel increases the risk of major bleeding to about 2% per year, a risk that will exist even if the daily dose of aspirin is reduced to 100 mg. Thus, the combination of clopidogrel and aspirin should only be used when there is a clear benefit. For example, combination therapy has not been shown to reduce the risk of acute ischemic stroke relative to clopidogrel alone or to reduce the risk of primary cardiovascular events when compared to aspirin alone.

As mentioned above, the onset of action of clopidogrel is slow, so even though platelet inhibition can be seen within a few hours after a single oral dose of the drug, a loading-dose between 300-600 mg is commonly given when prompt inhibition of the ADP receptors is desired, which is continued as a once daily oral dose of 75 mg for maintenance.

The documented adverse effects of clopidogrel include bleeding, severe neutropenia, and thrombotic thrombocytopenic purpura (TTP). Patients with a history of resolved aspirin-related peptic ulcers who received aspirin plus a PPI (e.g., esomeprazole) were shown to have a lower incidence of recurrence of peptic bleeding when compared to patients receiving clopidogrel instead. Another study suggested that prophylaxis with PPIs when undergoing treatment with clopidogrel following an acute coronary syndrome (ACS, i.e., unstable angina or MI) may increase the incidence of adverse cardiac events, perhaps as a result of the inhibition of the cytochrome P450 variant CYP2C19, which is required for the conversion of clopidogrel to its pharmacologically active form. However, even after some government health agencies issued a statement on a potential drug interaction between clopidogrel and PPIs, people within the cardiology community manifested concerns regarding the possible existence of flaws in the studies that served as the basis for these conclusions and subsequent warnings, putting into question the veracity of an adverse drug interaction between clopidogrel and PPIs.

Clopidogrel, was issued a black box warning from the FDA on March 12, 2010 because it is estimated that 2-14% of the US population have low levels of the CYP2C19 liver enzyme needed to activate clopidogrel and, therefore, may not get the full effect from the drug. However, there are tests available to predict if a patient will be susceptible to this reduced pharmacological effect.

3.2.2 Ticlopidine (Ticlid®)

Ticlopidine is an oral thienopyridine marketed under the trade name Ticlid by Roche Pharmaceuticals as 250 mg oral tablets.

Indications, dosage, and side effects

Ticlopidine is typically administered as an oral twice-daily dose of 250 mg. Like aspirin, ticlopidine is more effective than placebo at reducing the risk of cardiovascular death, MI, and stroke in patients with atherosclerotic disease, but due to its delayed onset of action, ticlopidine is not recommended for patients with acute MI. Ticlopidine has been routinely used in addition to aspirin after coronary artery stenting, and as a substitute for aspirin in patients with a contraindication to aspirin. However, because ticlopidine is less potent than clopidogrel and is associated with greater risk of hematologic disorders (e.g., neutropenia, TTP, thrombocytopenia, aplastic anemia), it has largely been replaced by clopidogrel. Due to the known hematologic side effects, which usually become manifest within the first few months of beginning therapy, frequent blood counts must be carefully performed when taking ticlopidine. As with clopidogrel, it is contraindicated in patients having hypersensitivity reactions to thienopyridines, as well as bleeding disorders, active bleeding, and liver disease.

3.2.3 Prasugrel (Effient®)

Prasugrel is an oral thienopyridine marketed under the trade names Effient, Efient, Apagrel, and Prasita. It was developed by Daiichi Sankyo Co. and is currently marketed in the United States in cooperation with Eli Lilly and Co. as 5 mg and 10 mg oral tablets.

Indications, dosage, and side effects

Prasugrel was approved for patients with acute coronary syndrome who will be undergoing a percutaneous coronary intervention (PCI) to reduce the occurrence of cardiovascular thrombotic events. Prasugrel is faster than clopidogrel at inhibiting ADP-induced platelet aggregation and does so to a greater extent than both normal and higher doses of clopidogrel in healthy individuals, as well as in patients with coronary artery disease, including those undergoing PCI. Unlike clopidogrel, prasugrel has not been shown to produce a lesser effect in patients who have a low level of hepatic CYP2C19 enzyme. Prasugrel should be administered as a single 60 mg oral loading dose and then continued at a dose of 10 mg orally once daily. Patients should also take aspirin (75-325 mg) per day.

A study published in the New England Journal of Medicine that compared prasugrel with clopidogrel in patients with acute coronary syndromes, both in combination with aspirin, found that prasugrel was a more potent anti-platelet agent, demonstrating a 1.2-fold reduction in the combined rate of cardiovascular mortality, nonfatal myocardial infarction, and nonfatal stroke. However, prasugrel was associated with a 1.6-fold rate of serious bleedings and 4-fold rate of fatal bleedings, even though overall mortality did not differ between the two patient groups.

3.2.4 Ticagrelor (Brilinta®)

Ticagrelor is an oral cyclopentyltriazolopyrimidine (CPTP) agent marketed under the trade names Brilinta, Brilique, and Possia. The drug was approved for use in the European Union on December 3, 2010 and by the US Food and Drug Administration on July 20, 2011, being marketed in the United States by AstraZeneca as 90 mg oral tablets.

In contrast to the other antiplatelet drugs clopidogrel, ticlopidine, and prasugrel, ticagrelor is a reversible allosteric inhibitor that does not require hepatic activation, making it a better choice for patients with hepatic insufficiency or those carrying low levels or genetic variants of the CYP2C19. Due to its reversible mode of action, ticagrelor is both faster and shorter acting than clopirogrel, making it a easier to discontinue (e.g., surgery, hypersensitivity), but typically requiring more frequent dosing, which can present an issue with compliance.

In a study by AstraZeneca, ticagrelor was associated with ~2% lower mortality rate than clopidogrel in patients with ACS and it was found that taking ticagrelor displayed a lower mortality rate from vascular causes, heart attack, or stroke. However, patients taking ticagrelor was associated with 1.5% higher propensity of non-lethal bleeding.

Indications, dosage, and side effects

Treatment with ticagrelor should be initiated as an oral loading dose of 180 mg, and then continued at 90 mg orally twice daily. Patients should also take aspirin (75-100 mg) daily. Ticagrelor is indicated for the prevention of thrombotic events in patients with ACS or MI, in combination with aspirin unless the latter is contraindicated. Compared with clopidogrel, ticagrelor significantly reduces the mortality rate in patients with ACS. The drug is contraindicated in patients with hepatic insufficiency and a history of pathological bleeding. It also should not be given in combination with other drugs that affect the CYP3A4 liver enzyme, since the drug is metabolized by CYP3A4 and is mainly excreted via bile and feces.

The most common side effects of ticagrelor are dyspnea as well as bleeding (e.g., gastrointestinal, nasal, subcutaneous/dermal). To date, less than 1% of patients taking ticagrelor have reported allergic reactions.

Inhibitors of hepatic CYP3A4 enzyme (e.g., ketoconazole and (?) grapefruit juice), increase blood plasma levels of ticagrelor and can therefore cause bleeding and other adverse effects. Conversely, activators of hepatic CYP3A4 (e.g., rifampicin and (?) St. John's wort), can reduce the effectiveness of ticagrelor. Furthermore, drugs that are also metabolized by CYP3A4 (e.g., simvastatin), will display higher plasma levels, which can result in an increase of the side effects of these drugs when combined with ticagrelor.

3.2.5 Thienopyridine resistance

There is variability among different individuals in the ability of the thienopyridines to inhibit ADP-induced platelet aggregation. To a certain extent this variability reflects genetic polymorphisms in the CYP isoenzymes associated with the metabolic activation of these drugs. For example, individuals carrying the CYP2C19*2 allele have been shown to display a lower responsiveness to clopidogrel, in a similar fashion as those having a lower activity of hepatic CYP3A4. These observations have resulted in the proposal that genetic testing may lead to the identification of individuals that may experience resistance to the effects of thienopyridines.

3.3 Phosphodiesterase inhibitors and adenosine reuptake inhibitors

As the name implies, phosphodiesterase inhibitors interfere with the function of the enzyme phosphodiesterase, which breaks down the intracellular second messenger cyclic adenosine monophosphate (cAMP). This results in increased levels of cAMP, ultimately leading to the inhibition of platelet activation and vasodilation.

3.3.1 Cilostazol (Pletal®)

Cilostazol is an oral phosphodiesterase inhibitor marketed under the trade name Pletal. The drug is marketed in the United States by Otsuka Pharmaceutical Co. as 50 and 100 mg oral tablets. Cilostazol is not used in the treatment of ischemic heart disease but rather in the relief of intermittent claudication in patients with peripheral vascular disease.

3.3.2 Dipyridamole (Persantine® and Aggrenox® (in combination with aspirin))

Dypyridamole is an oral phosphodiesterase inhibitor marketed as a single drug under the trade name Persantine, and as an extended-release combination with low-dose aspirin under the name Aggrenox. Persantine drug is marketed in the United States by Boehringer Ingelheim Pharmaceuticals, Inc. as 25, 50, and 75 mg oral tablets, while Aggrenox contains 200 mg of extended-release dipyridamole and 25 mg of aspirin.

Dypiridamole also inhibits the reuptake of adenosine by platelets, red blood cells, and vascular endothelial cells, as well as the enzyme adenosine deaminase, which metabolizes adenosine into inosine. Both of these effects increase the extracellular concentration of adenosine, which causes smooth muscle relaxation and is, at least in part, responsible for the vasodilatory effects of dipyridamole. Persantine causes vasodilation when given at high doses over a short time and it inhibits thrombosis when given long term by also acting as a thromboxane synthase inhibitor.

Indications, dosage, and side effects

The recommended dose of dipyridamole is 75-100 mg four times daily as an adjunct to warfarin therapy. Dipyridamole is a relatively weak antiplatelet agent on its own and thus is not used for the treatment of IHD. However, dipyridamole has been shown to increase myocardial perfusion and left ventricular function in patients with ischemic cardiomyopathy. In combination with low-dose aspirin (i.e., Aggrenox) it is used for prevention of stroke in patients with a history of transient ischemic attacks given as a twice-daily dose.

When given by intravenous infusion over 3-5 minutes, dipyridamole is associated with a rapid increase in the local concentration of adenosine in the coronary circulation, which has a vasodilatory effect. However, this vasodilation largely occurs in healthy coronary arteries, while those arteries that are stenosed remain so. This results in an imbalance of coronary perfusion that can become clinically manifest by symptoms of chest pain as well as electrocardiographic signs of ischemia.

Dipyridamole combined with aspirin reduces the risk of stroke by 22.1% compared with aspirin and by 24.4% compared with dipyridamole alone in patients with a history of cerebrovascular disease (i.e., TIA and/or stroke). With regard to secondary prevention in patients with a history of ischemic stroke, combination therapy resulted in 13% of patients having vascular death, stroke, or MI as opposed to 16% of those treated with aspirin alone. Based on all this data, Aggrenox is often used for stroke prevention. However, because it has vasodilatory effects, combination therapy of dipyridamole with aspirin (i.e., Aggrenox) should not be used for the prevention of stroke in patients with symptomatic coronary artery disease. A triple therapy of aspirin, clopidogrel, and dipyridamole has been investigated, but an increase in adverse bleeding events was observed with this combination.

The major side effects documented with the use of dipyridamole are gastrointestinal, headache, facial flushing, dizziness, and hypotension, which often disappear with continued use of the drug.

3.4 GP IIb/IIIa receptor antagonists

As a member of the integrin family of adhesion receptors, GP IIb/IIIa is found on the surface of platelets and megakaryocytes. With about 80,000 copies, GP IIb/IIIa is the most abundant receptor on platelets. GP IIb/IIIa consists of a non-covalently linked heterodimer that is inactive on resting platelets. When platelets are activated, a signal transduction pathway triggers a conformational change on the receptor that leads to its activation. Activated GP IIb/IIIa can bind other adhesion molecules (e.g., fibrinogen, vWF) under conditions of high shear stress. Binding is mediated by an Arg-Gly-Asp (RGD) sequence found on both fibrinogen and vWF, and by a Lys-Gly-Asp (KGD) sequence located within a unique dodecapeptide domain on fibrinogen. Once GP IIb/IIIa is bound to fibrinogen and/or vWF, adjacent platelets can be bridged together and lead to platelet aggregation.

Abciximab, eptifibatide, and tirofiban all target the GP IIb/IIIa receptor, but as described below, they are structurally and pharmacologically distinct. Abciximab has a long half-life and can be detected on the surface of platelets for a couple of weeks, while eptifibatide and tirofiban have shorter half-lives.

All of the GP IIb/IIIa antagonists are administered by intravenous (IV) infusion following an IV bolus. The dosage of eptifibatide and tirofiban must be reduced in patients with renal insufficiency since they are cleared by the kidneys.

The most serious complications of GP IIb/IIIa inhibitors are bleeding and thrombocytopenia, which is immunoglobulin-mediated as a result of antibodies directed against neoantigens on GP IIb/IIIa that form upon binding of the drug.

3.4.1 Abciximab (ReoPro®)

Abciximab is manufactured by Centocor and distributed by Eli Lilly. As with all of the GP IIb/IIIa antagonists, it is administered by intravenous (IV) infusion. It is a humanized murine monoclonal immunoblogulin Fab fragment directed against the activated form of GP IIb/IIIa that binds to the activated receptor with high affinity and blocks the binding of adhesion molecules.

Indications, dosage, and side effects

Abciximab is used in the setting of percutaneous coronary interventions (e.g., angioplasty, with or without stenting) to prevent platelet aggregation and thrombosis. It is administered as an IV bolus at 0.25 mg/kg, 10 to 60 min before PCI followed by continuous infusion of 0.125 µg/kg/min (to a max of 10 µg/min) for 12 h. Its use is associated with a reduction in both the incidence of ischemic complications, as well as the necessity for repeated interventional procedures within the first thirty days. Patients with diabetes and chronic renal insufficiency can be given abciximab, but its use is contraindicated in patients who shall be undergoing an emergent surgical procedure (e.g., coronary artery bypass grafting), since bleeding time may remain elevated for up to 12 hours.

Abciximab has a relatively short half-life (i.e., ~10-30 min), but its pharmacological effects on platelet function persist for up to 48 hours after cessation of IV infusion, followed by a low degree of GP IIb/IIIa receptor blockade that can continue for up to two weeks.

Many of the side effects of abciximab are due to its anti-platelet effects, including an increased risk of bleeding (e.g., gastrointestinal hemorrhage). Thrombocytopenia is a rare but known serious risk that occurs in up to 5% of individuals receiving the drug, which can be severe in ~1% of these patients. Abciximab-induced thrombocytopenia can typically be treated with transfusion of platelets. Abciximab induced thrombocytopenia can last for seven days after initial drug administration. Transfusing platelets is the only known treatment and may have limited effectiveness as the drug may also bind to the new platelets. Platelet counts, which should average 250,000-400,000, can effectively drop to zero.

In addition to targeting the GP IIb/IIIa receptor, abciximab also inhibits the closely related v3 receptor, which binds vitronectin, and M2, a leukocyte integrin. In contrast, eptifibatide and tirofiban are specific for GP IIb/IIIa. Inhibition of v3 and M2 may impart abciximab with anti-inflammatory and/or antiproliferative properties that extend beyond the inhibition of platelets.

3.4.2 Tirofiban (Aggrastat®)

Tirofiban is marketed the United States by Medicure Pharma and the rest of the world by Irokocardio International SARL under the brand name Aggrastat as a parenteral solution for intravenous administration in dosages of forms 5 mg and 12.5 mg. Tirofiban is a non-peptidic tyrosine derivative that mimics the RGD motif found on the ligands of GP IIb/IIIa.

Indications, dosage, and side effects

Tirofiban is administered intravenously with an initial dose of 0.4 µg/kg/min for the first 30 minutes, followed by a maintenance dose of 0.1 µg /kg/min as a constant IV infusion for 12-24 hours following PCI. Tirofiban, in combination with aspirin and heparin, is indicated in the treatment of patients with acute coronary syndromes (i.e., unstable angina or acute MI), including those who may be undergo subsequent percutaneous coronary intervention, to reduce the occurrence of further ischemic damage, new myocardial infarction, and mortality.

Tirofiban has a fast onset and short duration of action, with coagulation parameters returning to normal within 4-8 hours after intravenous infusion is stopped.

The major side effect of tirofiban seen in clinical trials was bleeding, both locally and systemically, with major bleeding occurring in 1.4% of patients and minor bleeding in 10.5%. About 4.0% of patients needed a transfusion to stop intractable bleeding and to improve anemia secondary to it. Thrombocytopenia was seen in patients given tirofiban and heparin at a rate of about 1.5%, compared to only 0.8% in those receiving heparin alone. This side effect was usually reversible within a few days. Positive fecal and urine hemoglobin tests were also seen. After the drug entered the market, there have been reports of intracranial and retroperitoneal bleeding, pulmonary hemorrhage, spinal-epidural hematoma, and hypersensitivity reactions including acute anaphylaxis. Fatal bleedings have been rarely reported.

3.4.3 Eptifibatide (Integrilin®)

Eptifibatide is a cyclic heptapeptide that binds GP IIb/IIIa because it contains the KGD motif. It is manufactured by Millennium Pharmaceuticals and co-promoted by Schering-Plough/Essex. Eptifibatide is supplied as a sterile solution in 10-mL vials containing 20 mg of the drug, and 100-mL vials containing either 75 mg or 200 mg of eptifibatide.

Indications, Dosage, and Side Effects

The recommended adult dosage of eptifibatide in patients with acute coronary syndrome that have normal renal function is an intravenous bolus of 180 µg/kg as soon as possible following diagnosis, followed by a continuous infusion of 2.0 µg/kg/min for up to 72 hours until hospital discharge or initiation of coronary artery bypass graft (CABG) surgery. For patients who are to undergo a percutaneous coronary intervention (PCI) while receiving eptifibatide, the infusion should be continued up to hospital discharge, or for up to 18 to 24 hours after the procedure, whichever comes first, allowing for up to 96 hours of therapy.

Eptifibatide is used to reduce the risk of acute cardiac ischemic events (i.e., death and/or myocardial infarction) in patients with unstable angina or non-ST-segment elevation (i.e., non-Q-wave) myocardial infarction (i.e., non-ST-segment elevation acute coronary syndromes) both in patients who are to receive non surgery (conservative) medical treatment and those undergoing percutaneous coronary intervention (PCI). The drug is always applied together with aspirin or clopidogrel and (low molecular weight or unfractionated) heparin.

The side effects of eptifibatide are very similar to those of abciximab.

4. Ongoing trials of antiplatelet therapy

According to the International Committee of Medical Journal Editors (ICMJE):

"Any research study that prospectively assigns human participants or groups of humans to one or more health-related interventions to evaluate the effects on health outcomes."

Over the past ten years, government agencies and the IMCJE have issued laws and directives on the subject of trial registration. All parties have consistently agreed that the purpose of trial registration is to promote the public good by ensuring that the existence and design of clinically directive trials are publicly available. The registration effort began with the development of a publicly available website, ClinicalTrials.gov, which is a service of the NIH, developed by the National Library of Congress.

In 1997, the FDA/NIH began requiring registration for only a limited number of trials. In September, 2007, the Food and Drug Amendments Act (Title VIII. Sec. 801) significantly expanded the scope of clinical trials that must be registered. Penalties for failing to register "applicable trials" may include civil monetary penalties.

In 2004, the International Committee of Medical Journal Editors (ICMJE) defined trials that must be registered in order to be considered for publication in journals that adhere to ICMJE standards. In 2007 the ICMJE expanded the definition of trials that must be registered. Scores of journals (not limited to medical journals) have adopted the registration policy.

The best way to obtain information about clinical trials in platelet activation in ischemic heart disease is by accessing two renowned sources:

http://clinicaltrials.gov

http://www.clinicaltrialresults.org/

Clinicaltrials.gov is a site organized by US government and their webpage states:

"ClinicalTrials.gov offers up-to-date information for locating federally and privately supported clinical trials for a wide range of diseases and conditions. A clinical trial (also clinical research) is a research study in human volunteers to answer specific health questions."

ClinicalTrials.gov currently contains 112,970 trials sponsored by the National Institutes of Health, other federal agencies, and private industry. Studies listed in the database are conducted in all 50 States and in 175 countries. ClinicalTrials.gov receives over 50 million page views per month and 65,000 visitors daily.

The U.S. National Institutes of Health (NIH), through its National Library of Medicine (NLM), has developed this site in collaboration with the Food and Drug Administration (FDA), as a result of the FDA Modernization Act, which was passed into law in November 1997. See the FDA document - Guidance for Industry: Information Program on Clinical Trials for Serious or Life-Threatening Diseases and Conditions (March 2002).

This site allows for selection of all important characteristics of clinical trial to be displayed. We can choose any combination of next characteristics: condition, intervention, sponsor, gender, age group, phase, number enrolled, funded by, study type, study design, NCT ID, other IDs, first received date, start date, completion date, last updated date, last verified date, acronym, primary completion date, and outcome measure.

The second site, http://www.clinicaltrialresults.org/, can be used as excellent source of slides, movies, reports, and other useful information about clinical trials. The 'cardiology' section contains divisions into subspecialty news, with listing about: acute coronary syndromes, angina, anticoagulants, antiplatelet agents, antithrombins, congestive heart failure, electrophysiology, imaging, interventional cardiology, prevention, and patient resources. Since access to these sources is in the public domain, we decided not to cite individual trials by other sources although we went deeper and extracted information from from individual trials. We advise our readers to visit these two sites frequently.

A reasonably informative overview of ongoing trials of antiplatelet therapy is supposed to list name and registry number for trial, to describe study population, specify primary end point, and define study arms. This data is presented in table 4.1

Clinical Trial (Registry No.)	Study Population	Primary End Point	Study Arms
ACCOAST (NCT01015287)	4,100 patients with NSTEMI planned to undergo PCI	CV death, MI, stroke, urgent revascularization, or GP IIb/IIIa inhibitor bailout at 7 days	Randomized to pre-treatment with prasugrel (30 mg at time of diagnosis with additional 30 mg atPCI) vs. prasugrel (60 mg) at PCI. Maintenance therapy in both arms will be 10 mg daily with dose reduction to 5 mg in patients >75 yrs and body weight <60 kg
ARCTIC (NCT00827411)	2,500 patients undergoing elective PCI with DES	Death, MI, stroke, urgent coronary revascularization, or stent thrombosis assessed at 1 yr; death, MI, stroke, urgent coronary revascularization, or stent thrombosis at 6–18 months after second randomization	Initial randomization to tailored antiplatelet therapy with VerifyNow P2Y12 vs. standard dual antiplatelet therapy. Subsequent randomization after 12 months of patients who remain eventfree to discontinuation of antiplatelet therapy or continuation of therapy
DANTE Trial (NCT00774475)	442 patients with NSTE-ACS undergoing PCI with stent implantation found to have high residual platelet reactivity with the VerifyNow P2Y12	CV death, MI, or target vessel revascularization at 6 months and 1 yr	Randomized to 75 mg of clopidogrel or 150 mg of clopidogrel
DAPT (NCT00977938)	20,645 subjects undergoing PCI	CV death, MI, and stroke at 33 months; stent thrombosis at 33 months	Subjects in the overall cohort who are free from death, MI, stroke, repeat revascularization, stent thrombosis, or major bleeding at 12 months will be randomized to 18 additional months of dual antiplatelet therapy or aspirin and placebo

Clinical Trial (Registry No.)	Study Population	Primary End Point	Study Arms
GRAVITAS (NCT00645918)	2,783 subjects after DES placement for stable CAD or NSTE-ACS will have platelet function testing done with VerifyNow P2Y12	CV death, MI, and definite/ probable stent thrombosis at 6 months	Patients with high residual platelet reactivity will be randomized to receive standard-dose clopidogrel (75 mg daily) or high-dose clopidogrel (600 mg load, 150 mg daily). A random sample of patients without high residual platelet reactivity will also be enrolled and will receive 75 mg of clopidogrel daily
INNOVATE-PCI (NCT00751231)	Phase II trial in 800 patients undergoing elective PCI	No pre-specified primary end point	Randomized to clopidogrel (300/600 mg load, followed by 75 mg daily) or elinogrel (80 mg IV bolus administered before PCI, followed by twice daily dosing of oral 50 mg, 100 mg, or 150 mg)
LANCELOT 201 (NCT00312052)	Phase II trial of 600 patients with CAD	Safety and tolerability (6 months)	Randomized to E5555 (50 mg, 100 mg, or 200 mg daily) or placebo
LANCELOT 202 (NCT00548587)	Phase II trial of 600 patients with CAD	Safety and tolerability (12 weeks)	Randomized to E5555 (50 mg, 100 mg, or 200 mg daily) or placebo
TRA-CER (NCT00527943)	12,500 subjects with ACS	CV death, MI, stroke, recurrent ischemia with repeat hospital stay, and urgent coronary revascularization at end of study	Randomized to SCH 530348 (40 mg loading dose, 2.5 mg daily) vs. placebo
TRA-2P-TIMI 50 (NCT00526474)	26,450 patients with history of CAD, CVA, or PAD	CV death, MI, stroke, and urgent coronary revascularization at end of study	Randomized to SCH 530348 (2.5 mg daily) vs. placebo
TOPAS-1 (NCT00914368)	Phase II trial of 450 patients who have either had or not had stent thrombosis or MI within 6 months of PCI while on dual antiplatelet therapy	Establish VerifyNow P2Y12 (PRU) and VASP (PRI, %) cutoff level of platelet inhibition in patients with and without clinical events.	All subjects will undergo platelet function testing with both VerifyNow P2Y12 and VASP assays

Clinical Trial (Registry No.)	Study Population	Primary End Point	Study Arms
TRIGGER-PCI (NCT00910299)	2,150 subjects with high residual platelet reactivity with the VerifyNow P2Y12 after elective PCI with DES	CV death or MI at 6 months	Randomized to prasugrel (60 mg load, 10 mg daily) vs. clopidogrel (75 mg daily)
TRILOGY-ACS (NCT00699998)	10,300 patients with NSTE-ACS being initially medically managed	CV death, MI, or stroke at end of study	Randomized to prasugrel (30 mg load ifadministered, followed by 5 mg or 10 mg maintenance) or clopidogrel (300 mg load if administered, followed by 75 mg daily)

Table 4.1

5. Abbreviations

ACCOAST: Comparison of Prasugrel at PCI or Time of Diagnosis of Non-ST Elevation Myocardial Infarction Trial

ACS: acute coronary syndrome

ARCTIC: Double Randomization of a Monitoring Adjusted Antiplatelet Treatment Versus a Common Antiplatelet Treatment for DES Implantation, and Interruption Versus Continuation of Double Antiplatelet Therapy Trial

ARMYDA: Antiplatelet Therapy for Reduction of Myocardial Damage During Angioplasty

CIPAMI: Clopidogrel Administered Prehospital to Improve Primary PCI in Patients with Acute Myocardial Infarction

CAD: coronary artery disease

CLARITY-TIMI: Clopidogrel as Adjunctive Reperfusion Therapy-Thrombolysis in Myocardial Infarction

CREDO: Clopidogrel for the Reduction of Events During Observation

CURE: Clopidogrel in Unstable Angina to Prevent Recurrent Events

CURRENT/OASIS: Clopidogrel Optimal Loading Dose Usage to Reduce Recurrent Events/Optimal Antiplatelet Strategy for Interventions

CV: cardiovascular

CVA: cerebrovascular accident

DANTE: Dual Antiplatelet Therapy Tailored on the Extent of Platelet Inhibition

DAPT: Dual Antiplatelet Therapy

DES: drug-eluting stents

GP IIb/IIIa: glycoprotein IIb/IIa

GRAVITAS: Gauging Responsiveness With A VerifyNow Assay—Impact On Thrombosis And Safety

INNOVATE-PCI: A Phase 2 Safety and Efficacy Study of PRT060128, a Novel Intravenous and Oral P2Y12 Inhibitor, in Non-Urgent PCI

LANCELOT 201: Safety and Tolerability of E5555 and Its Effects on Markers of Intravascular Inflammation in Subjects With Coronary Artery Disease

LANCELOT 202: Safety and Tolerability of E5555 and Its Effects on Markers of Intravascular Inflammation in Subjects With Acute Coronary Syndrome

MI: myocardial infarction

NSTE-ACS: non–ST-segment elevation acute coronary syndrome

NSTEMI: non–ST-segment elevation myocardial infarction

PAD: peripheral artery disease

PCI: percutaneous coronary intervention

PRI: platelet reactivity index

PRINCIPLE: Prasugrel in Comparison to Clopidogrel for Inhibition of Platelet Activation and Aggregation

PRU: platelet reactivity unit

STEMI: ST-segment elevation myocardial infarction

TIMI: Thrombolysis In Myocardial Infarction

TOPAS-1: Tailoring Of Platelet Inhibition to Avoid Stent Thrombosis

TRA-CER: Trial to Assess the Effects of SCH 530348 in Preventing Heart Attack and Stroke in Patients With Acute Coronary Syndrome

TRA-2P-TIMI 50: Trial to Assess the Effects of SCH 530348 in Preventing Heart Attack and Stroke in Patients With Atherosclerosis

TRIGGER-PCI: Testing Platelet Reactivity In Patients Undergoing Elective Stent Placement on Clopidogrel to Guide Alternative Therapy With Prasugrel

TRILOGY-ACS: Comparison of Prasugrel and Clopidogrel in Acute Coronary Syndrome Subjects

TRITON: Trial to Assess Improvement in Therapeutic Outcomes by Optimizing Platelet Inhibition with Prasugrel

VASP: Vasodilator-stimulated phosphorprotein

6. References

Antman, E. M. & Loscalzo, J. (2012). Chapter 245. ST-Segment Elevation Myocardial Infarction, In: *Harrison's Principles of Internal Medicine, 18e,* Fauci, A. S., Braunwald E., Kasper D. L., Hauser S. L., Longo D. L., Jameson J. L., & Loscalzo J., McGraw-Hill, Retrieved from http://www.accessmedicine.com/content.aspx?aID=9104591.

Antman, E. M., Selwyn, A. P., & Loscalzo, J. (2012). Chapter 243. Ischemic Heart Disease, In: *Harrison's Principles of Internal Medicine, 18e,* Fauci, A. S., Braunwald E., Kasper D. L., Hauser S. L., Longo D. L., Jameson J. L., & Loscalzo J., McGraw-Hill, Retrieved from http://www.accessmedicine.com/content.aspx?aID=9104321

Antoniades, C., Shirodaria, C., Van Assche, T., Cunnington, C., Tegeder, I., Lötsch, J., Guzik, T. J., Leeson, P., Diesch, J., Tousoulis, D., Stefanadis, C., Costigan, M., Woolf, C. J., Alp, N. J., & Channon, K. M. (2008). GCH1 haplotype determines vascular and plasma biopterin availability in coronary artery disease effects on vascular superoxide production and endothelial function. *J. Am. Coll. Cardiol.,* Vol. 52, pp. 158-165.

AstraZeneca (22 August 2011). BRILINTA™ (ticagrelor) tablets now available in U.S. pharmacies for patients with acute coronary syndrome, In: *http://www.astrazeneca-us.com/,* Available from: http://www.astrazeneca-us.com/search/?itemId=12475851

AstraZeneca (August 2011). Brilinta, In: *http://www.astrazeneca-us.com/our-medicines/,* Available from: http://www1.astrazeneca-us.com/pi/brilinta.pdf

Banga, H. S., Simons, F. R., Brass, L. F., & Rittenhouse, S. E. (1986). Activation of phospholipases A and C in human platelets exposed to epinephrine: role of glycoproteins IIb/IIIa and dual role of epinephrine. *Proc. Natl. Acad. Sci.,* Vol. 83, pp. 9197-9201.

Bassenge, E. (1996). Endothelial function in different organs. *Progress in Cardiovascular Diseases,* Vol. XXXIX, No. 3, pp. 209-228.

Beckman, J. S. & Koppenol, W. H. (1996). Nitric oxide, superoxide, and peroxynitrite: the good, the bad, and ugly. *Am. J. Physiol.,* Vol. 271, pp. C1424-C1437.

Bonauer, A., Boon, R. A., & Dimmeler, S. (2010). Vascular microRNAs. *Curr. Drug Targets,* Vol. 11, No. 8, pp. 943-949.

Brass, L. F. (1984). The effect of Na^+ on Ca^{2+} homeostasis in unstimulated platelets. *J. Biol. Chem.,* Vol. 259, pp. 12571-12575

Brass, L. F. (2010). Understanding and Evaluating Platelet Function Hematology. *Am. Soc. Hematol. Educ. Program.,* pp. 387-396

Cannon, C. P. & Braunwald, E. (2012). Chapter 244. Unstable Angina and Non-ST-Segment Elevation Myocardial Infarction, In: *Harrison's Principles of Internal Medicine, 18e,* Fauci, A. S., Braunwald, E., Kasper, D. L., Hauser, S. L., Longo, D. L., Jameson, J. L., & Loscalzo, J., McGraw-Hill, Retrieved from http://www.accessmedicine.com/content.aspx?aID=9104518 clinicaltrials.gov: http://clinicaltrials.gov/ct2/results?flds=Xt&flds=a&flds=b&term=Antiplatelet+Therapy&show_flds=Y

Cooley, H. & Cohen, P. (1968). Potassium transport in human blood platelets. *J. Lab. Clin. Med.,* Vol. 70, pp. 69-79.

Dousset, J., Trouilh, M., & Fogliett, M. (1983). Plasma malonaldehyde levels during myocardial infarction. *Clinica. Chimica. Acta*, Vol. 129, pp. 319-322.

Edelstein, L. C. & Bray, P. F. (2011). MicroRNAs in platelet production and activation. *Blood*, Vol. 17, No. 20, pp. 5289-5296.

Enauf, J., Bredoux, R., Bourdeau, N., & Levy, S. (1987). Two different Ca^{2+} transport systems are associated with plasma and intracellular human platelet membranes. *J. Biol. Chem.*, Vol. 262, pp. 9293-9297.

Fang, Y., Shi, C., Manduchi, E., Civelek, M., & Davies, P. F. (2010). MicroRNA-10a regulation of proinflammatory phenotype in athero-susceptible endothelium in vivo and in vitro. *Proc. Natl. Acad. Sci. USA*, Vol. 107, No. 30, pp. 13450-13455.

Frojmovic, M. & Panjwani, R. (1976). Geometry of normal mammalian platelets by quantitative microscopic studies. *Biophys. J.*, Vol. 16, pp. 1071-1089.

Garelnabi, M. (2010). Emerging Evidences from the Contribution of the Traditional and New Risk Factors to the Atherosclerosis Pathogenesis. J. Med. Sci., Vol. 10, pp. 136-144.

Garelnabi, M., Gupta, V., Mallika, V., & hattacharjee, J. (2010). Platelets oxidative stress in Indian patients with ischemic heart disease. *J. Clin. Lab. Anal.*, Vol. 24, No. 1, pp. 49-54.

Garelnabi, M., Gupta, V., Mallika, V., & Bhattacharjee, J. (2011). Platelet Nitric Oxide Signaling System in Patients with Coronary Artery Disease. *Ann. Vasc. Dis.*, Vol. 4, No. 2, pp. 99–105.

Hagemeyer, C. E. & Peter, K. (2010). Targeting the platelet integrin GP IIb/IIIa. *Curr. Pharm. Des.*, Vol. 16, No. 37, pp. 4119-4133.

Haver, V. G., Slart, R. H., Zeebregts, C. J., Peppelenbosch, M. P., & Tio, R. A. (2010). Rupture of vulnerable atherosclerotic plaques: microRNAs conducting the orchestra? *Trends Cardiovasc. Med.*, Vol. 20, No. 2, pp. 65-71.

Heptinstall, S. & Hanley, S. (1985). Blood platelets and vessel walls, In: *Hemostasis and Thrombosis, 1st Ed.*, pp. 36-74, Butterworths, USA.

Hourani, M. & Lausck, J. (1991). Pharmacological Receptors on Blood Platelets. *Pharmacol. Rev.*, Vol. 43, pp. 243-298.

Ikeda, H., Takajo, Y., Murohara, T., Ichiki., K., Adachi, H., & Haramaki, N. (2000). Platelet-derived nitric oxide and coronary risk factors. *Hypertension*, Vol. 35, pp. 904–907.

Jamaluddin, M. S., Weakley, S. M., Zhang, L., Kougias, P., Lin, P. H., Yao, Q., & Chen, C. (2011). miRNAs: roles and clinical applications in vascular disease. *Expert Rev. Mol. Diagn.*, Vol. 11, No. 1, pp. 79-89.

Karpatkin, S., Charmatz, A., & Langer, M. (1970). Glycogenesis and glyconeogenesis in human platelets. Incorporation of glucose, pyruvate, and citrate into platelet glycogen, glycogene synthetase and fructose-1,6-diphosphate activity. *J. Clin. Invest.*, Vol. 49, pp. 140-149.

Knezevie, I., Dieter, P., & Le Breton, C. (1992). Mechanism of inositol 1,4,5-triphosphate-induced aggregation in saponin-permeabilized platelets. *J. Pharmacol. Exp. Ther.*, Vol. 260, pp. 947-955.

Leeper, N. J., Raiesdana, A., Kojima, Y., Chun, H. J., Azuma, J., Maegdefessel, L., Kundu, R. K., Quertermous, T., Tsao, P. S., & Spin, J. M. (2011). MicroRNA-26a is a novel regulator of vascular smooth muscle cell function. *J. Cell. Physiol.*, Vol. 226, No. 4, pp. 1035-1043.

Leslie, V., Christel, B., Patricia, J., & Ulhas, N. (1999). Platelets in Hemostasis and thrombosis, In: *Wintrobe's Clinical Hematology, 10th Edition,* Vol. 1, pp. 661-683, Williams & Wilkins, Maryland, USA.

Malmgren, R. (1986). ATP-Secretion occurs as an initial response in collagen induced platelet activation. *Thromb. Res.,* Vol. 43, pp. 445-453.

Nurden, A. T. (2011). Platelets, inflammation and tissue regeneration. *Thromb. Haemost.,* Vol. 105, Suppl. 1, pp. S13-S33.

O'Sullivan, J. F., Martin, K., & Caplice, N. M. (2011). Microribonucleic acids for prevention of plaque rupture and in-stent restenosis: "a finger in the dam". *J. Am. Coll. Cardiol.,* Vol. 57, No. 4, pp. 383-389.

Pan, Z. W., Lu, Y. J., & Yang, B. F. MicroRNAs: a novel class of potential therapeutic targets for cardiovascular diseases. *Acta Pharmacol. Sin.,*Vol. 31, No. 1, pp. 1-9

Parthasarathy, S. Litvinov, D. Selvarajan, K., Garelnabi, M. (2008). Lipid peroxidation and decomposition – conflicting roles in plaque vulnerability and stability, *Biochimica et Biophysica Acta,* Vol. 1781, pp. 221–231.

Paulus, M., Bur, J., & Grosdent, C. (1979). Control platelet territory development in megakaryocytes. *Blood Cells,* Vol. 5, pp. 59-88.

Petidis, K., Douma, S., Doumas, M., Basagiannis, I., Vogiatzis, K., & Zamboulis, C. (2008). The interaction of vasoactive substances during exercise modulates platelet aggregation in hypertension and coronary artery disease. *BMC Cardiovasc. Disord.,* Vol. 27, No. 8, pp. 11.

Selwyn, A. P., & Braunwald, E. (1994). Ischemic Heart disease. In: *Harrison's Principles of Internal Medicine, 13th Ed.,*Vol. 1, pp. 1077, McGraw-Hill, Inc. New York, USA.

Siess, W., Cautrecasas, P., & Lapetina, G. (1983). A role for cyclooxygenase products in the formation of phosphatidic acid in stimulated human platelets. Differential mechanism of action of thrombin and collagen. *J. Biol. Chem.,* Vol. 258, pp. 4683-4686.

Siess, W. (1989). Molecular mechanism of platelet activation. *Physiol. Rev.,* Vol. 69, pp. 58-177.

Siljander, P. R. M. Platelet-derived microparticles–an updated perspective. (2011). *Thrombosis Research,* Vol. 127, Suppl. 2, pp. S30-S33

Smith, B., Ingerman, C., Kocsis, J., & Silver, M. (1973). Formation of prostaglandins during aggregation of human blood platelets. *J. Clin. Invest.,* Vol. 52, pp. 965-969.

Stenberg, E., Shuman, A., Levine, P., & Bainton, F. (1984). Redistribution of alphagranules and their contents in thrombin-stimulated platelets. *J. Cell Biol.,* Vol. 98, pp. 748-760.

Urbich, C., Kuehbacher, A., & Dimmeler, S. (2008). Role of microRNAs in vascular diseases, inflammation, and angiogenesis. *Cardiovasc. Res.,* Vol. 79, No. 4, pp. 581-588.

Weiss, J., Kelly, A., & Herbert, V. (1968). Vitamin B_{12} and folate activity in normal human platelets. *Blood,* Vol. 31, pp. 258-262.

Weitz, J. I. (2012). Chapter 118. Antiplatelet, Anticoagulant, and Fibrinolytic Drugs, In: *Harrison's Principles of Internal Medicine, 18e,* Fauci, A. S., Braunwald, E., Kasper, D. L., Hauser, S. L., Longo, D. L., Jameson, J. L., Loscalzo J., McGraw-Hill, Retrieved from http://www.accessmedicine.com/content.aspx?aID=9101027

Weksler, B. B. (1983) Platelets and the inflammatory response. *Clin. Lab. Med.,* Vol. 3, No. 4, pp. 667-76.

WHO (2008). The World Health Report 2008: Primary Health Care Now More Than Ever. World Health Organization, Geneva, Switzerland, p. 119.

Wierda, R. J., Geutskens, S. B., Jukema, J. W., Quax, P. H., & van den Elsen, P.J. (2010). Epigenetics in atherosclerosis and inflammation. *J. Cell. Mol. Med.*, Vol. 14, No. 6A, pp. 1225-40.

Wikipedia (21 August 2011). Antiplatelet drug, In: *http://en.wikipedia.org/*, 5 September 2011, Available from: http://en.wikipedia.org/wiki/Antiplatelet_drug (including all links and references cited within).

Zehnder, J. L. (2009). Chapter 34. Drugs Used in Disorders of Coagulation, In: *Basic & Clinical Pharmacology, 11e*, Katzung, B. G., Masters, S. B., Trevor, A. J., pp. 598-600, McGraw-Hill, ISBN 978-0-07-160405-5, New York, NY, USA

Zhenyu, L., Delaney, M. K., O'Brien, K. A., & Du, X. (2010). Signaling During Platelet Adhesion and Activation. *Arterioscler. Thromb. Vasc. Biol.*, Vol. 30, pp. 2341-2349.

9

Myocardial Ischemia-Reperfusion/Injury

Nermine Saleh and Magda Youssef
Faculty of Medicine, Ain Shams University, Physiology Department
Egypt

1. Introduction

Refers to myocardial, vascular, or electrophysiological dysfunction that is induced by the restoration of blood flow to previously ischemic tissue. Tissue damage caused when blood supply returns to the tissue after a period of ischemia. The absence of oxygen and nutrients from blood during the ischemic period creates a condition in which the restoration of circulation results in inflammation and oxidative damage through the induction of oxidative stress rather than restoration of normal function.

Early reperfusion of ischemic myocardium is an accepted approach for the management of patients with acute coronary syndromes. In addition, surgical interventions requiring interruption of blood flow to the heart, out of necessity, must be followed by restoration of perfusion. Reperfusion, although essential for tissue and/or organ survival, is not without risk due to the extension of cell damage as a result of reperfusion itself.

Since rupture of the plasma membrane is a prominent feature of necrosis and ischemia-reperfusion injury and is a lethal event, it is worth considering what might lead to rupture of the plasma membrane. Rupture of the plasma membrane could be facilitated by calpain or some other protease cleavage of the cytoskeleton. Complete loss of ATP would also inhibit ion pumps, which would result in swelling perhaps rupturing the plasma membrane, particularly if the cytoskeleton has been weakened (Murphy & Steenbergen, 2008).

It is possible that a combination of protease activation with loss of ATP, ion dysregulation and cell swelling all conspire to rupture the plasma membrane. A rise in cytosolic free Ca^{2+} concentration $[Ca^{2+}]_i$ has been consistently observed in ischemia and early reperfusion. A rise in $[Ca^{2+}]_i$ will lead to activation of calpains, which could be involved in cleaving proteins leading to plasma membrane rupture. Calpain activates the proapoptotic BID, and also cleaves Atg5, shifting the balance from autophagy to apoptosis. An increase in $[Ca^{2+}]_i$ and ROS can lead to activation of an inner mitochondrial large-conductance channel known as the Mitochondrial permeability transition (MPT). Opening of this channel would lead to loss of ATP and mitochondrial function, which would quickly lead to mitochondrial swelling and release of cytochrome *c*, which could activate apoptosis. If a large number of mitochondria in a cell undergo opening of the MPT, the cell will lose the capacity to make ATP, and the cell will lose ion homeostasis, resulting in cell swelling, membrane rupture, and cell death (Murphy & Steenbergen, 2008).

Platelet-dependent thrombus formation is a key event in the pathogenesis of acute myocardial infarction (AMI). Platelets mediate both thrombotic occlusion of the entire epicardial coronary artery and also accumulate in the microcirculation resulting in impairment of microcirculation and provoking myocardial ischemia during reperfusion (Gawaz, 2004)..

Despite an improved understanding of the pathophysiology of this process and encouraging preclinical trials of multiple agents, most of the clinical trials to prevent reperfusion injury have been disappointing. Despite these problems, adjunctive therapies to limit reperfusion injury remain an active area of investigation. In these studies vitamin E has been tried to ameliorate lethal reperfusion injury.

2. Protective effects of vitamin E against myocardial ischemia/reperfusion injury in rats

Prevention of ischemia-reperfusion (I/R) injury is crucial for successful cardiac surgery. In cardiac surgery, it is reported that pharmacological agents can be administered prior to ischemia, enabling them to exert their protective effects on mitochondria prior to ischemia and reperfusion. The role of α-tocopherol (vitamin E) as a chain-breaking antioxidant is well characterized in vitro; it is considered the major lipophilic antioxidant in the human body, specifically by its reaction with peroxyl free radicals (Navarro et al., 2005). It has been demonstrated that vitamin E deficiency is responsible for increased myocardial injury caused by oxidative stress and that I/R of the heart is associated with a blunting in cardiac α-tocopherol levels (Altavilla et al., 2000). Vitamin E has been extensively assayed in experimental animal diseases, and in the protection and treatment of human diseases.

Research provided evidence that vitamin E intake much higher than the current recommended dietary allowance could contribute to or improve human health. It has been reported that dietary requirements to prevent deficiency and maintain apparent health is substantially less than optimal amounts necessary to provide protection against degenerative conditions and chronic diseases. Results of a number of studies suggested that increased vitamin E intake is associated with decreased risk of coronary heart disease, and certain types of cancer as well as enhancement of immune function (Ricciarelli et al., 2002 ; Dong et al., 2009). Literatures concerning safety, and tolerance of oral vitamin E demonstrated that vitamin E is relatively nontoxic (Dong et al., 2009; Hanson et al., 2007). In a 91-day study of rats receiving up to 316-443 mg vitamin E/animal/day, vitamin E had no adverse effects on weight gain, food intake, organ weights, hematology or serum chemistry values (Krasavage et al., 1977). In the heart and cardiovascular system, nitric oxide (NO) plays a significant role. The specific roles of NO in the heart in general and on cardiac mitochondria in particular remain controversial. It has been reported that both endogenous and exogenous sources of NO exert important modulatory effects on mitochondrial function (Davidson & Duchen, 2006). Nitric oxide donors have been shown to induce a powerful cardioprotection against I/R injury in mice (Wang et al., 2005). However, literature reporting varying results of NO therapy, with some investigators reporting cardioprotective effects, whereas others report cardiotoxic effects (Bell et al., 2003). Mitochondrial permeability transition (MPT) is a nonspecific pore in the inner mitochondrial membrane. It has been reported that the opening of the MPT converts the mitochondria from an organelle that provides adenosine triphosphate to sustain heart function into an instrument of cell death by apoptosis if the insult is mild, and to necrosis if the insult is profound (Halestrap et al., 2004). It is hypothesized that a major component of I/R injury is necrotic cell death, which is widely thought to be the consequence of opening the MPT as reported by previous literature (Costa et al., 2006). Functional recovery of the Langendorff-perfused heart from ischemia inversely correlates with the extent of the opening, and inhibition of the MPT provides protection against reperfusion injury (Halestrap et al., 2004). Previous literature (Kim et al., 2006) reported that radical oxygen species (ROS) generated during early reperfusion is the primary activator of the MPT, and cardiomyocyte death. Some recently developed, intracellularly targeted scavengers have been reported to provide some reduction in infarct size (Sheu et al., 2006). Antioxidants such as vitamins C, and E have also been suggested to scavenge ROS and reduce ischemic injury (Qin et al., 2006). A study, therefore, was performed with the following objectives, first, to determine whether a short course of oral administration of vitamin E in a megadose as compared to a NO donor nitroglycerin (GTN) can provide sufficient protection of the heart against reperfusion induced injury, and second, to determine whether a combined regimen of vitamin E and a NO donor confound superior protection to the hearts against this insult, and to investigate the effect of each of these pharmacological preconditioning agents on mitochondria and MPT.

2.1 Methods

This study was undertaken on female Wistar rats weighing 150-200 gm. Rats were allocated into 4 groups: a- Control group, non-treated , b- GTN-treated group, rats received GTN intraperitoneal 25 minutes before sacrifice, in a dose of 120 μg/kg bw (Zhou et al., 2002) ,c- Vit E-treated group, rat received vitamin E by oral tubal feeding 16-20 hours before sacrifice, in a dose of 250mg/rat d- Vit E and GTN-treated group, rats received vitamin E and GTN as in both GTN-treated group and vit E -treated group.

Experimental procedures; On the day of the experiments, rats were weighed and injected intraperitoneally with heparin sodium, 1000 IU. One hour later, the rats were anesthetized with thiopental sodium 40 mg/kg intraperitoneally.

In vitro studying of isolated hearts: Hearts were excised and perfused in a Langendorff preparation with the standard Krebs-Henselite Bicarbonate (KHB) buffer, pH 7.4 equilibrated with $O_2:CO_2$ (95%:5%) at 37 ° C (Ayobe &Tarazi, 1983). After 20 minutes stabilization period, baseline cardiac activities were recorded using isometric force transducer connected to a two-channel oscillograph.

Ischemia Reperfusion Technique:: After recording baseline cardiac activity, 30 minutes of ischemia was induced by stopping the perfusing fluid, and at 30-minute reperfusion, the cardiac activity was recorded again.

Cardiac activity was assessed by the following parameters: heart beating rate (BR), rate of tension development (dT/dt) and half relaxation time (1\2 RT). Myocardial flow rate (MFR) was measured at the same intervals by timed volumetric collection. Results were expressed as the percentage change of the measured parameters relative to baseline values to normalize individual differences between basal values among each group.

The cardiac chambers were weighed. The ventricles were used to isolate mitochondria. Mitochondria were isolated by conventional procedures of differential centrifugation. Hydrolysis of mitochondrial nicotinamide adenine dinucleotide (NAD $^+$) directly reflects MPT opening. The NAD$^+$ was measured after perchloric acid extraction (Di Lisa et al., 2001; Yamazaki et al., 2004). The malondialdehyde (MDA) was estimated in cardiac homogenates by the double heating method of Draper and Hadley (Draper & Hadley, 1990). Data for MDA and NAD$^+$ was calculated by non-parametric Mann –Witney test.

Electron microscopic study: Parts of the lower half of the left ventricle were fixed in 4% glutaraldehyde, dehydrated and embedded in resin. Sections of 60 nm thickness were cut on copper grids and stained with uranyl acetate followed by lead citrate for examination by the electron microscope (Hunter, 1984).

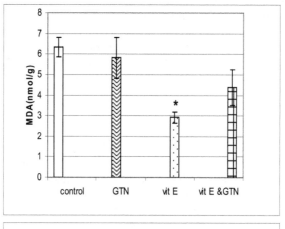

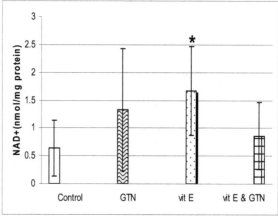

Fig. 1. The malondialdehyde (MDA) and mitochondrial nicotinamide adenine dinucleotide (NAD $^+$) levels after 30 minutes reperfusion in control rats, nitroglycerine-treated rats (GTN), vit E-treated rats and vit E & GTN-treated rats. Data are presented as means ± SD *
P = 0.004 as compared to control rats.

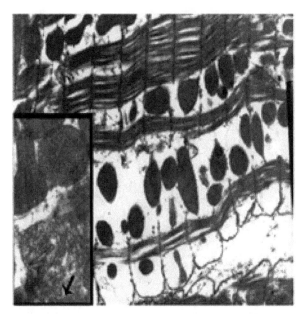

Fig. 2. Showing irregular, disorted myofilaments. They appear loose and discontinuous.Mitochondiae are pleomorphic and idely spaced (controll group x60000). Arrow shows disruption in the mitochondrial membrate (x15000).

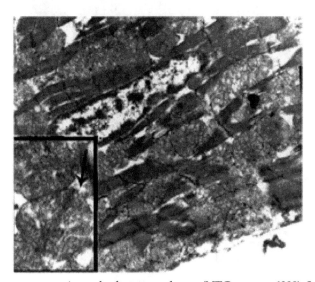

Fig. 3. Myofilaments appear irregular but more dense. (NTG group x6000). Inset – mitochondriae show disrupted cristae and arrow shows discontinuous mitochondrial membrane (x15000). GTN group – group received nitroglycerin

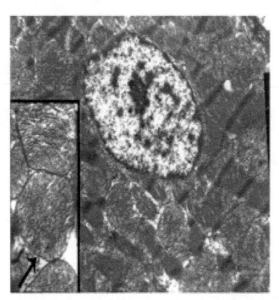

Fig. 4. Showing regular dense and continuous myofilaments. (Vit E group x6000). Inset – mitochondriae are regular in shape. They reveal transverse, parallel cristae.Arrow shows continuous mitochondrial membrane. (x15000). Vit E group – received vitamin E.

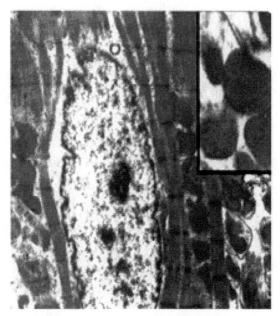

Fig. 5. Showing regular and dense myofilaments (GTN and Vit E group x6000.). Inset – mitochondriae are electron dense with unclear cristae. (x15000). GTN and Vit E group – received nitroglycerin and vitamin E.

Group (n=7)	%BR	%dT/dt	%½RT	%MFR
Control	-16.21±4.93	-23.75±6.88	22.85±9.84	-21.78±13.07
GTN-tr.	-21.16±11.04	22.94±20.64	46.43±19.57	-53.31±9.74
Vit E-tr.	15.37±26.21	39.66±24.43[a]	10.71±12.02	-17.57±17.68[b]
Vit E and GTN-tr.	-15.10±7.11	38.48±23.67[a]	14.29±5.04	-25.44±4.24

Data are presented as mean ± SEM. n: is the number of rats. a:Significance calculated by least significant difference (LSD) at P=0.03 from control group, b:Significance calculated by LSD at P=0.04 between vit E-tr., and GTN-tr groups. BR - beating rate, dT/dt - rate of tension development, ½ RT -half relaxation time, MFR - myocardial flow rate.

Table 1. Percentage changes from baseline values of cardiac activity at 30 minutes reperfusion after 30 minutes of ischemia (I/R) of perfused hearts isolated from; control rats, GTN-treated rats (GTN-tr.),vitamin E-treated rats (vitE-tr.), and vitamin E & nitroglycerin-treated rats (vit E and GTN-tr.).

2.2 Effects of vitamin E versus nitroglycerine on I/R injury

Our results demonstrated that a short course of vitamin E treatment induced preconditioning in the hearts. The vitamin E therapy, enhanced contractile, and vascular recovery, and attenuated oxidative stress in cardiac tissue, as demonstrated by the decrease of MDA in cardiac tissue. Moreover, this therapy protected the hearts against MPT opening as indicated by significant increase of NAD$^+$ in cardiac tissue. Histological examination showed less mitochondrial injury induced by reperfusion in the hearts of this group, with preservation of the myocytes structure. Moreover, the present study clearly demonstrated that preischemic treatment with GTN; a NO donor did not provide significant protection of hearts against I/R-induced contractile dysfunction and tissue injury. Peroxynitrite (ONOO-), the reacting product of NO and O_2^-, is apotent cytotoxic agent. It is highly reactive with a wide variety of molecules, including deoxyribose, cellular lipids, and protein sulfhydryls, and results in oxidative tissue damage (Farshid et al., 2002). In this study, GTN treatment did not attenuate the reperfusion-mediated increase of MDA in cardiac tissues of GTN-treated rats. This finding suggested that ONOO- might be formed excessively in post-ischemic myocardial tissue. In the current study, supplementation of NO donor could have raised cardiac tissue NO concentration, with the coincident increase in free radical generation at reperfusion established the conditions of ONOO- formation. Therefore, we suggest that exogenous NO failed to provide cardioprotection, due to concomitant increase of ONOO-. In this study, the non significant increase of NAD$^+$ content in isolated hearts from GTN-supplemented rats indicated failure of GTN to attenuate MPT opening. The opening of that channel lead to mitochondrial swelling, release of apoptotic molecules and eventually cell death. This suggestion was further confirmed by histological examination of isolated hearts from GTN-supplemented rats. Previous literature (Dhalla et al., 2000) reported a depletion of endogenous antioxidants in the ischemic hearts upon reperfusion. Various studies have reported the beneficial effects of antioxidants as these agents render resistance to the hearts against I/R injury. However, other investigators have failed to observe such results. The slow incorporation of vitamin E into tissues, due to its marked lipophilicity, is probably responsible for its failure as a cardioprotective compound as shown during the acute administration of α-tocopherol after

I/R injury induced in the pig (Altavilla et al., 2000). Several studies reinforce the importance of localization and timing in cardioprotection. Delivery of the antioxidants to the right compartment in the right time period is very difficult to achieve in controlled animal studies, and even more difficult in patients. As a result of the controversy in the animal studies, and the failed clinical trials, it is often concluded that inhibition of ROS will not influence infarct size. A more realistic assessment is that to have a significant benefit in reducing infarct size requires the correct delivery of mitochondrial targeted antioxidants perhaps in conjunction with other therapies. So in this study, we tried to give the animals vitamin E in a large dose, with a sufficient time to provide its effects. The demonstration that prior exposure to a low concentration of H_2O_2 protects against MPT opening may be of pathophysiological importance for cardioprotection (Costa et al., 2006). By the same reasoning, in preconditioning, we speculate the need for an antioxidant that attenuates the large burst of oxidative stress at the start of reperfusion without completely neutralizing free radicals.

We suggest that vitamin E as a physiological antioxidant acted to scavenge free radicals without completely neutralizing them, thereby affording a significant preconditioning effect. Reduction of free radical formation inhibits MPT opening, thereby affording preconditioning. This is clearly demonstrated in the current study, since there was a significant increase of NAD+ content of reperfused hearts in the vitamin E-treated groups. Histological examination confirmed this result, as it revealed marked protection of the normal structure of myocytes and mitochondria. Addition of GTN treatment to vitamin E attenuated its cardioprotective effect. In summary, the findings of the present study provide evidence that a short course of vitamin E treatment protected the heart against reperfusion-injury compared to a NO donor. The MPT is an important target of this protection.

3. Effects of vitamin E treatment on age-associated changes in cardiac responses to the injury of post I/R

Aging is one of the most important risk factors for the development of cardiovascular disease. Aging is characterized by loss of myocytes, remodeling and impaired contractile function in the heart. The rate of programmed cell death in the left ventricle increases with age (Kwak et al., 2006). Meanwhile the aged heart faces a high risk of free radical injury owing to slow generation of antioxidant enzymes by its cells, and a general decline in this system may be another reason for the development of myocardial dysfunction (Asha Devi et al., 2003 a).

It is well established that nitric oxide (NO), is constitutively generated within the heart, not only by the endothelium but also by the myocytes (Balligand et al., 1995). Numerous previous animal studies have reported that there is a loss of NO biological activity and /or biosynthesis during aging (Matz et al., 2000).

Oxygen free radicals increase in concentration upon reperfusion of ischemic cardiac tissue (Xia et al., 1996). It is well established that these reactive species can interact with and damage various cellular components (Berlett & Stadtman, 1997). Free radical production in the heart has also been reported to increase with age (Sohal et al., 1990). Thus, although restoration of blood flow is the sole method for salvaging ischemic tissue, oxidative damage may occur during reoxygenation and contribute to ischemia–reperfusion injury.

Regular exercise is a key component of cardiovascular risk prevention strategies. Physical activity is known to cause generation of free radicals. Exercise training in old animals failed to enhance antioxidant activity (Hatao et al., 2006). However swim training especially at low-intensity, was found to be beneficial as a major protective adaptation against oxidative stress particularly in the older myocardium (Kiran et al., 2004). The tocopherols (major vitamers of vitamin E) are believed to play a role in the prevention of human aging-related changes, and are of particular interest, mainly because of their antioxidative properties (Asha Devi et al., 2003 b).

From the aforementioned data, it seems possible that free radical - mediated injury is a major issue in the increase of aging related reperfusion-induced myocardial dysfunction. Exercise training program could not always protect the aging heart satisfactorily. We tried to test the hypothesis that using an antioxidant as vitamin E could lead to better protection of the aging hearts as compared with exercise training.

Therefore, a study was conducted to compare the effects of vitamin E treatment versus swim- exercise training on age- associated changes in cardiac responses to the injury of post I/R.

3.1 Methods

This work was undertaken on female Wistar rats aged 16-18 months. Rats were allocated into 3 groups: a) Control group of aged rats, b) Exercise -trained aged rats subjected to daily physical exercise by swimming in the water tank, for 2 hours daily, 6 days aweek for 2 weeks, and c) Vitamin E-treated aged rats subjected to daily injection of vitamin E (300 mg/kg) intraperitoneally, 6 days aweek for 2 weeks.

The swim-training program adopted was according to Refaat et al., (1989), in a swimming tank, filled with water and maintained at thermoneutral temperature of 30°c. A motor fan in the tank stirs strong water currents. This ensures uniformity of temperature and forces the rats to swim actively all the time.

3.1.1 Experimental procedures

They were done as previously described (Ayobe &Tarazi, 1983). Peak developed tension per left ventricular weight as well as coronary flow rate per left ventricular weight were calculated relative to left ventricular weight (PT/LV, g /100mg)& (CF/LV, ml /100mg/min).

Nitrate concentration in coronary effluents, as a stable product of nitric oxide (NO), was measured by an endpoint one-step enzymatic assay using nitrate reductase, as described by Bories and Bories, (1995), and modified in tissues by Kassim, (1997).

3.1.2 Effects of exercise on cardiac weights and post Ischemia-reperfusion (I/R) responses

In this study, exercise was found to exert a trophic effect on cardiac chambers manifested by significant increase of the absolute & relative weights of atria, right ventricle, and left ventricle. Swimming is well recognized for its effectiveness in inducing myocardial hypertrophy (Evangelista et al., 2003). Exercise can protect cardiac function of the aging heart by protection against; loss of cardiac myocytes, reduction in number of myonuclei, reactive hypertrophy of remaining myocytes, and increased connective tissue in left ventricle (LV) of the aging rat heart. This protection is achieved through attenuation of age-

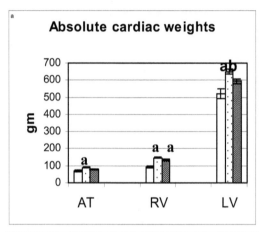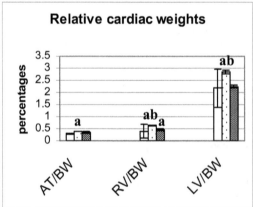

induced elevation in Bax/Bcl-2 ratio, thereby inhibits apoptosis (Asha Devi et al., 2003a), and exerts its trophic effect.

Although exercise-trained rats had significant increase in LV and LV/BW that indicates LV hypertrophy, they showed Peak developed tension similar to control which could be attributed to the increase of free radical in aged rats induced by exercise. Oxygen free radicals are known to have deleterious effects on contractile force of heart (Gao et al., 1996).

Fig. 6. Mean values± SEM of: absolute weights (mg) of atria (AT), right ventricle (RV), left ventricle (LV), and their relative weights (mg/g) (AT/BW), (RV/BW), (LV/BW) in control rats ☐ , exercise-trained rats ⬚ , and vit. E-treated rats ▩ .
a.   Significance calculated by least significant difference (LSD) at P < 0.05 from control group.
b.   Significance calculated by LSD at P < 0.05 between vit E-treated, and exercise-trained groups

The results of ischemia-reperfusion of isolated hearts from both control and exercise-trained aged rats have shown the lack of tolerance to ischemia-reperfusion injury as regard inotropic activities as well as myocardial flow rate. This could be explained in view of the increase in free radicals generation induced by exercise, even if small, was added to the increased free radicals generation induced by aging exceeding the antioxidant defense capacity of the heart leading to loss of beneficial cardio-protective effect of exercise on ischemia-reperfusion injury (Hatao et al., 2006).

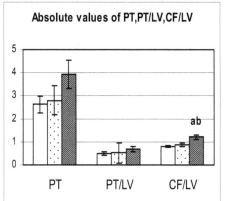

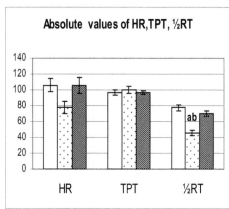

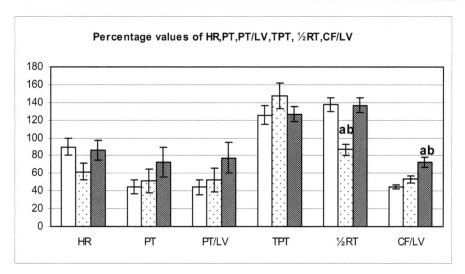

Fig. 7. Mean absolute and percent values ± SEM of: heart beating rate(HR), Peak developed tension(PT), Peak developed tension per left ventricular weight(PT/LV), Time to peak tension (TPT), Half relaxation time(½ RT), and Coronary flow rate per left ventricular weight (CF/LV), at 30 minutes reperfusion of hearts isolated from control rats ☐ , exercise-trained rats ⬚ , and vit. E- treated rats ▨ .

a. Significance calculated by least significant difference (LSD) at $P < 0.05$ from control group.
b. Significance calculated by LSD at $P < 0.05$ between vit E-treated, and exercise-trained groups

The increased free radicals generation such as superoxide anion could react with NO to form peroxynitrate, decreasing NO biological activity. Peroxynitrate molecule by itself might play a significant role in oxidative tissue damage. This is supported in this study by the absence of increase of nitrates in the coronary effluent from exercise- trained aged rats at 30 min reperfusion.

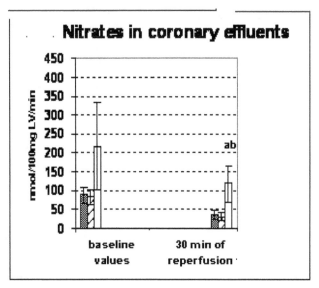

Fig. 8. Mean values ±SEM of nitrates in coronary effluents (nmol/100mg LV/min) at baseline values, and 30 minutes of reperfusion in control rats ▓, exercise-trained rats ▨, and vit. E-treated rats ☐.
a. Significance calculated by least significant difference (LSD) at P < 0.05 from control group.
b. Significance calculated by LSD at P < 0.05 between vit E-treated, and exercise-trained groups

Also, the heart beating rate of the exercise-trained rats could not be preserved after 30 min of reperfusion. This could be attributed to the increased free oxygen radicals in these rats, since oxyradicals have been implicated as a possible cause of reperfusion arrhythmias (Tanguy et al., 1998). However, the rate of relaxation of hearts excised from exercise-trained rats showed better tolerance to I/R after initial intolerance, and such improvement is in accordance to a recent report by Libonati et al., (2005), who found that sprint training in rats improves post-ischemic left ventricular diastolic stiffness due to up-regulation of myocardial glycolysis, with ATP production that protects the heart from ischemia-reperfusion as it plays an important role in actin-myosin rigor bond dissociation, and regulating myocardial diastolic function.

Effects of vitamin E on cardiac weights and Post Ischemia-Reperfusion (I/R) responses:

Vitamin E has been reported to stimulate upregulation at the expression level of B cl-2 gene, B cl-2 molecule is involved in the inhibition of apoptosis (Azzi et al., 2004).

Therefore, vitamin E by preventing apoptosis of myocardial cells could be expected to induce hypertrophy of the heart (trophic effect). However in case of vitamin E–treated rats, results have shown that the effect of vitamin E on the rate of growth of right and left ventricles was not similar. While the rate of growth of right ventricle was increased by the anti-apoptosis effects of vitamin E. The increase in left ventricle & left ventricle/ body weight was insignificant. This could be attributed to the favorable effects of vitamin E on reduction of blood pressure and blood viscosity (Costa et al., 2005). These two factors have been claimed to induce growth of left ventricle during aging (Ghali et al., 1997). Thereby, by eliminating these two factors, the rate of growth of left ventricle was decreased under the influence of vitamin E supplementation counteracting its trophic effect in aged rats.

In contrast to aged control rats and exercise-trained aged rats, the isolated hearts from vitamin E-treated rats showed better tolerance as regard inotropic activity, especially force generation measured as peak developed tension as well as coronary flow rate. In accordance, Venditti et al., (1999) showed a protective action of vitamin E treatment against lipid peroxidation and cardiac dysfunction associated with ischemia- reperfusion in rats. Vitamin E decreases free radical deleterious effect on cell membrane, proteins, DNA, and decreases both ROS mediated direct ischemia-reperfusion mediated injury, as well as peroxynitrite-mediated injury and thereby preserving NO through preventing its inactivation by its transformation to peroxynitrite (Kamat, 2006). In support, this study showed significant increase of nitrates in coronary effluent from vitamin E- treated aged rats measured at 30 min of reperfusion.

In view of the aforementioned data, vitamin E proved to be a cardio-protective agent as it attenuated the injury of post ischemia-reperfusion on the aged myocardium. This beneficial effect of vitamin E could be partially attributable to preservation of NO biological activity by preventing its transformation to the toxic compound peroxynitrite.

On the other hand, the swim-training program adopted in this study, as regard tolerance to ischemia-reperfusion apart from improvement of half relaxation time, the swim-training program did not show other promising cardio-protective effects against cardiac changes associated with the aging process.

Therefore, vitamin E supplementation could be recommended to aged people especially patients suffering from ischemic heart disease. Vitamin E could be used either alone or in combination with exercise training taking into consideration the duration and intensity of exercise program.

Vitamin E and platelet function

Platelets play a critical role in the pathophysiology of reperfusion (Gawaz, 2004). Platelet function is not static during ischemia-reperfusion. Instead, during ischemia regional platelet aggregability is increased. Systemic and regional platelet aggregability also increases during myocardial reperfusion. The mechanism of these responses is unknown but may be related to regional endothelial dysfunction created by ischemia. The response observed could also be explained by the release of proaggregatory mediators in the coronary and/or systemic circulation during ischemia-reperfusion (Gurbel et al., 1995).

Reperfusion induces an important inflammatory response, characterized by a massive production of free radicals and by the activation of the complement and leucocyte neutrophils (Gourdin et al., 2009). Platelets and neutrophils act synergistically in provoking postreperfusion cardiac dysfunction (Lefer et al., 1998). Activated platelets play an important role in the process of myocardial ischemia-reperfusion injury, and platelet-derived P-selectin is a critical mediator (Xu et al., 2006), whereas platelet P-selectin promotes platelet interactions with leukocytes. Because platelets release potent proinflammatory chemokines and modulate leukocyte function, platelet accumulation in the postischemic microvasculature might significantly contribute to the manifestation of I/R injury (Massberg et al., 1998).

Reperfusion of the tissue, subsequent to ischemia, results in burst of oxygen consumption with consequent generation of oxygen derived free radicals; the oxidant-anti oxidant status of the tissue is thrown out of balance and multi dimensional free radical mediated damage ensues. Since vitamin E is a potent natural anti-oxidant, its administration is expected to restore the imbalance.

Effect of administration of 600 mg vitamin E each day, for six days, was observed on activity of some of the anti-oxidant enzymes and levels of malondialdehyde (as an index of free radical mediated damage) in the platelets of patients reperfused after myocardial infarction. It has been found that vitamin E administration significantly lowers the level of malondialdehyde in the patients. Vitamin E administration increases the activities of anti oxidant enzymes (superoxide dismutase, glutathione reductase and catalase) tested both in the patients and healthy controls. However, lowering of lipid peroxidation upon administration of vitamin E is specific for patients. These findings exhibit beneficial role of vitamin E administration in the management of the patients reperfused after myocardial infarction (Dwivedi et al., 2005).

The results of Chen et al, (2002) suggested that the reduction of myocardial I/R injury with vitamin E supplementation may be the result of the inhibition of polymorphonuclear neutrophil (PMN) CD11b expression.

Vitamin E supplementation in healthy subjects or patients with hypercholesterolemia was shown to diminish platelet function as assessed by ex vivo platelet aggregation of 11-dehydrothromboxane B_2, a marker of in vivo platelet activation (Calzada et al., 1997; Davi et al., 1997). Celestini et al., (2002) demonstrated that vitamin E can potentiate the antiplatelet activity of aspirin by inhibiting the early events of platelet activation pathway induced by collagen.

A study from our laboratory was to examine the possibility that vitamin E administration could exert an effect on blood elements and platelet aggregation.

Materials and Methods

Albino rats of both sexes weighing 180- 220 gm fed on a standard rat diet and fasted for 18-24 hours before sacrifice were used in this study.

In vivo study: A total of 30 rats were used in this study. They were divided in two groups. Group I: Saline control group; rats in this group were injected with saline instead of vitamin E, daily for 5 consecutive days. Group II: vitamin E treated group; rats were injected with vitamin E (300 mg/kg b.w.) intraperitoneally for five consecutive days. After 5 days all injections were stopped for 2 days. By the seventh day rats were anesthetized with pentobarbitone in a dose of 40 mg/kg b.w.

Collection of blood samples: blood samples were obtained by arterial puncture from the abdominal aorta. One ml samples were collected into tubes containing EDTA for examination of RBCs and platelet counts, hemoglobin content and hematocrite values.

Another blood samples were collected in chilled plastic tubes containing sodium citrate 3.8gm/100 ml (9 volumes of blood to 1 volume of sodium citrate) and gently shaken. These blood samples were used for study of platelet aggregation. The citrated blood was centrifuged at 1500 r.p.m. for 5 min. The supernatant platelet rich plasma (PRP) was pipetted into clean plastic tubes. The remaining blood sample was centrifuged at 10,000 r.p.m. for 10 min. to prepare platelet poor plasma (PPP). Standard PRP: the number of platelets in PRP was counted using coulter T-660 counter. The platelet number was adjusted to a standardized number of 3×10^5 platelet per µl by dilution with autologus platelet poor plasma.

Aggregation study: platelet aggregation was performed using Chrono-Log automatic aggregometer (model 540-VC, Chrono-Log Corp, Harvertown, USA) coupled with computer and printer. ADP as an aggregating agent was used at a final concentration of 10 uM. The maximum aggregation was recorded after 3 min.

In vitro of vitamin E on platelet aggregation

Collection of blood samples: blood was collected from normal rats, anaesthetized by pentobarbitone, by arterial puncture from abdominal aorta into chilled tubes containing sodium citrate 3.8 gm%. Preparation of standard PRP was carried out as described in the in vivo experiments.

The in vitro effect of vitamin E on ADP- induced platelet aggregation was studied by exposing PRP to rising concentrations of the vitamin 1,2,3,4 and 5 mg/ml. Equal volumes of saline were added to control samples.

Aggregation study: was carried as described above in vivo experiments.

Statistical analysis of the data was done using Student's "t" test for unpaired data according to Fisher and Yates (1957) $P < 0.05$ was considered significant.

Regression study: linear regression analysis was used to relate different parameters to a certain outcome (platelet aggregation) to find out the highest beta coefficient and the most important factor affecting this outcome. This analysis was performed on SPSS windows version eight.

Results

Table 1 portrays the results of in vivo effects of vitamin E on hematological parameters. RBCs count, Hb content and PCV showed slight and insignificant changes in vitamin E treated rats compared to their saline controls. The number of platelets was insignificantly decreased in vitamin E treated animals. However platelet aggregation induced by ADP showed a significant decrease ($P < 0.05$) in this group (table 2 and figure 9).

Regression analysis: as seen in fig. 10, multiple regression analysis of platelet aggregation against other parameters. Only a significant negative correlation between platelet number and platelet aggregation was seen in vitamin E treated group (P < 0.03).

In vitro effect of vitamin E on platelet aggregation: the platelet aggregation effect of ADP in presence of rising concentration of vitamin E showed significant inhibition (P <0.01) only when vitamin E was added at a final concentration of 5 mg/ml. Addition of vitamin E in smaller concentrations of 2- 4 mg/ml final concentration produced insignificant inhibition of platelet aggregation. Almost no effect was seen when vitamin E was added at a final concentration of 1 mg/ml (table 3 and figure 11).

Parameters / Group treatment	RBCs x 10^6/ul	Hb gm/dl	PCV %	Platelet count x 10^3/ul	Platelet aggregation %
Saline control (15)	6.54±0.3	12.24±0.5	36.15±1.2	1146±71.12	68.1±1.9
Vitamin E treated rats (15)	6.33±0.2	11.93±0.3	35.3±0.9	1068±53.1	58.9±4
P	NS	NS	NS	NS	< 0.05

Data are mean± SEM In parenthesis is the number of observations   NS: non significant

Table 2. Red blood cell count (RBCs), hemoglobin level (Hb), packed cell volume (PCV), platelet count and platelet aggregation in saline control and vitamin E treated rats.

Additions to normal PRP					
	Final concentration of vitamin E				
Saline control (12)	1mg/ml (8)	2mg/ml (9)	3mg/ml (11)	4mg/ml (11)	5mg/ml (13)
50.08±2.6	50.75±2	47.1±2.32	44.36±2.85	44.7±3.4	37.23±3
P	NS	NS	NS	NS	< 0.01

Data are mean± SEM In parenthesis is the number of observations NS: non significant

Table 3. In vitro effect of vitamin E on platelet aggregation of normal rat PRP in presence of different concentrations of vitamin E compared to saline control

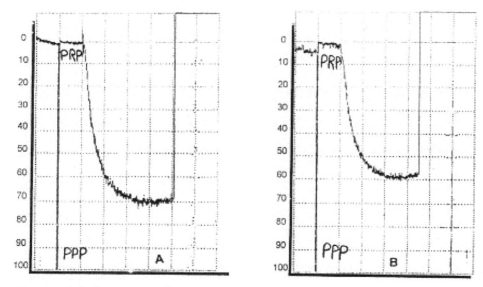

ADP-induced platelet aggregation%

Fig. 9. Tracing of ADP- induced platelet aggregation of Vitamin E-treated rats (B) compared to saline treated rats (A).

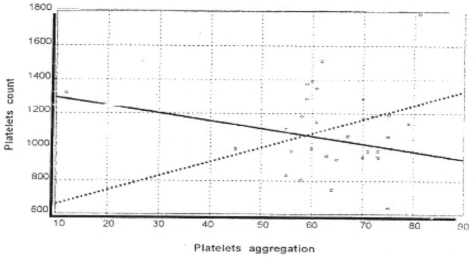

Vitamin E- treated rats ▬▬▬▬

Saline- treated rats ••••••••••••

Fig. 10. Correlation between platelet aggregation and platelet count among vitamin E-treated rats and saline treated rats (by multiple regression analysis)

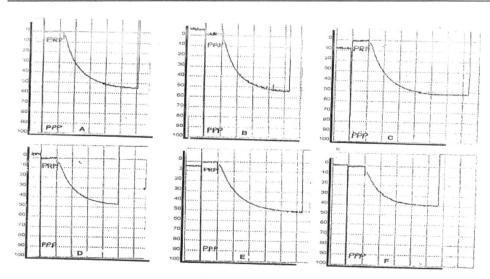

Fig. 11. Tracing of ADP- induced platelet aggregation of normal rats PRP in presence of vitamin E in concentrations of 1, 2, 3, 4 and 5 mg/ml respectively (B- F) compared to saline control (A)

The data reported here demonstrated that administration of megadose of vitamin E (300 mg/kg for one week) to rats, produced slight and nonsignificant changes in red blood cell counts, hemoglobin content, packed cell volume. Platelet counts showed an insignificant decrease. However, the platelet aggregation responses to ADP of PRP from treated rats were significantly inhibited. This finding shows the safety of vitamin E in this supra-physiological dose of 300 mg/kg on blood parameters tested.

On addition of vitamin E to normal PRP in vitro, the platelet aggregating effect of ADP showed significant inhibition only when vitamin E was added at a final concentration of 5 mg/ml. Addition of vitamin E in smaller concentrations of 2- 4 mg/ml produced insignificant inhibition of platelet aggregation. Almost no effect was seen when vitamin E was added at a final concentration of 1 mg/ml.

From these data, it can be concluded that this supra physiological dose of vitamin E is safe concerning the blood parameters tested.

The observation in the present study that vitamin E when added in vitro to normal rat PRP caused significant inhibition of platelet aggregation in response to ADP; illustrate that vitamin E by itself exerts a direct antiplatelet effect. Higashi & Kikuchi (1974) were the first to demonstrate that vitamin E inhibits the aggregation of platelets using hydrogen peroxide as the aggregating stimulus. Subsequent studies by Steiner & Anastasi, (1976) demonstrated that vitamin E also inhibited platelet aggregation response to epinephrine, collagen and ATP. Moreover, Freedman and Keaney, (2001) found that platelet incorporation of vitamin E both in vitro and in vivo leads to dose-dependent inhibition of platelet aggregation in response to agonists such as arachidonic acid and phorbol ester.

Although it is best known for its antioxidant activity the exact mechanism of the antiplatelet effect of vitamin E is not exactly known and one of the following mechanisms may operate. First, it can be attributed to altered metabolism of prostaglandins. The vascular generation of prostacyclin (PGI$_2$) is higher and the platelet thromboxane A$_2$ generation is lower than normal. This view is supported by the findings of Steiner and Anastasi (1976) and others (Karpen et al., 1981; Pritchard et al., 1982; Pignatelli et al., 1999) that vitamin E inhibits platelet thromboxane A$_2$ synthesis. On the other hand, PGI$_2$ synthesis is stimulated possibly by reduction of cellular peroxide level (Gilbert et al., 1983). Second, the inhibition of platelet aggregation can be explained by the ability of vitamin E to inhibit intracellular mobilization of sequestrated calcium from the dense tubular system of the cytoplasm (Srivastava, 1986). Third, by its membrane stabilizing action, vitamin E would impair platelet release reaction. This view is supported observations of Feki et al., (2001) that vitamin E by its antioxidant effect, protects molecules and tissue against the deleterious effect of free radicals and also contributes to the stabilization of biological membranes. Fourth, unrelated to its antioxidant action, vitamin E was shown to inhibit protein kinase C (PKC) in various cell types with consequent inhibition of platelet aggregation (Azzi et al., 2002; Freedman et al., 1996; Freedman and Keaney, 2001). Further, vitamin E includes inhibitory effects are the result of specific interactions with component of the cell e.g. proteins, enzymes and membranes (Ricciarelli et al., 2002).

Vitamin E attenuated P-selectin expression on activated human platelets and thus inhibited the P-selectin–dependent function, platelet–mononuclear cell (MNC) interaction. The mechanism probably was related to the inhibition of PKC activity in platelets. Since P-selectin is an important atherothrombogenic adhesion molecule, this finding will provide us new insights into the mechanism by which dietary vitamin E inhibits thrombosis and atherogenesis and thereby reduces the risk of coronary artery diseases (Murohara et al, 2004).

Although these studies from our laboratory have shown that vitamin E administered in megadose, could provide a protective effect against the cardiac responses to the injury of post I/R. Further studies should be conducted to test the possibility of using vitamin E in cardiac surgery.

4. References

Altavilla, D., Deodato, B., Campo, GM., Arlotta, M., Miano, M., Squadrito, G., Saitta, A., Cucinotta, D., Ceccarelli, S., Ferlito, M., Tringali, M., Minutoli, L., Caputi, AP. & Squadrito F. (2000). IRFI 042, a novel dual vitamin E-like antioxidant, inhibits activation of nuclear factor-kappaB and reduces the inflammatory response in myocardial ischemiareperfusion injury, *Cardiovasc Res* 47: 515-528.
Asha Devi, S., Prathima, S.& Subramanyam, MV. (2003 a). Dietary vitamin E and physical exercise: II, Antioxidant status and lipofuscin-like substances in aging rat heart, *Exp Gerontol.* 38: 291-297.
Asha Devi, S., Prathima, S.& Subramanyam, MV. (2003 b). Dietary vitamin E and physical exercise: I. Altered endurance capacity and plasma lipid profile in ageing rats, *Exp Gerontol.* 38: 285-290.

Ayobe, MH. & Tarazi, RC. (1983). beta-Receptors and contractile reserve in left ventricular hypertrophy, *Hypertension* 5: I192- I197.

Azzi, A., Gysin, R., Kempná, P., Munteanu, A., Negis, Y., Villacorta, L., Visarius, T.& Zingg, JM. (2004). Vitamin E mediates cell signaling and regulation of gene expression, *Ann N Y Acad Sci.* 1031:86-95.

Azzi, A., Ricciarelli, R. & Zingg, JM. (2002). Non-oxidant molecular functions of alpha-tocopherol
(vitamin E), *FFBS Lett.* 22: 519.

Balligand, JL., Kobzik, L., Han, X., Kaye, DM., Belhassen, L., O'Hara, DS., Kelly, RA., Smith, TW.& Michel, T. (1995). Nitric oxide-dependent parasympathetic signaling is due to activation of constitutive endothelial (type III) nitric oxide synthase in cardiac myocytes, *J Biol Chem.* 270(24):14582-14586.

Bell, RM., Maddock, HL.& Yellon, DM. (2003). The cardioprotective and mitochondrial depolarising properties of exogenous nitric oxide in mouse heart, *Cardiovasc Res* 57: 405-415.

Berlett, B S. & Stadtman E R. (1997). Protein oxidation in aging, disease, and oxidative stress, *J Biol Chem.*;272:20313–20316.

Bories, PN. & Bories C.(1995). Nitrate determination in biological fluids by an enzymatic one-step assay with nitrate reductase, *Clin. Chem.* 41: 904-907.

Calzada, C., Bruckdorfer, KR. & Rice-Evans, C.A. (1997). The influence of antioxidant nutrients on platelet function in healthy volunteers, Atherosclerosis. 128: 97.

Celestini, A., Pulcinelli, FM., Pignatelli, P., Frati, G., Gazzaniga, PP. & Viol,i F. (2002). Vitamin E potentiates the antiplatelet activity of aspirin in collagen-stimulated platelets, *Haematologica.* 87(4):420.

Chen, Y. , Davis-Gorman, G. , Watson, RR. & McDonagh, PF. (2002). Vitamin E attenuates myocardial ischemia-reperfusion injury in murine AIDS, *Cardiovasc Toxicol.* 2 (2): 119- 27.

Costa, AD., Jakob, R., Costa, CL., Andrukhiv, K., West, IC.& Garlid, KD. (2006). The mechanism by which the mitochondrial ATP-sensitive K+ channel opening and H2O2 inhibit the mitochondrial permeability transition, *J Biol Chem* 281: 20801-20808.

Costa, VA., Vianna, LM., Aguila, MB.& Mandarim-de-Lacerda, CA. (2005). Alpha-tocopherol supplementation favorable effects on blood pressure, blood viscosity and cardiac remodeling of spontaneously hypertensive rats, *J Nutr Biochem* . 16: 251-256.

Davi, G., Alessandrini, P., Minotti, MG, Bucciarelli, T., Costantini, F., Cipollone F., Bittolo Bon, G., Ciabattoni, G. & Patrono, C. (1997). In vivo formation of 8-epiprostaglandin F2a is increased in hypercholesterolemia, Arterioscler Thromb Vasc Biol. 17: 3230.

Davidson, SM. & Duchen, MR. (2006). Effects of NO on mitochondrial function in cardiomyocytes: Pathophysiological relevance, *Cardiovasc Res* 71: 10-21.

Dhalla, NS., Elmoselhi, AB., Hata, T.& Makino, N. (2000). Status of myocardial antioxidants in ischemia-reperfusion injury, *Cardiovasc Res* 47: 446-456.

Di Lisa, F., Menabò, R., Canton, M., Barile, M.& Bernardi, P. (2001). Opening of the mitochondrial permeability transition pore causes depletion of mitochondrial and cytosolic NAD+ and is a causative event in the death of myocytes in postischemic reperfusion of the heart, *J Biol Chem* 276: 2571-2575.

Dong, YH., Guo, YH. & Gu, XB. (2009). Anticancer mechanisms of vitamin E succinate, *Chin J Cancer* 28: 1114-1118.

Draper, HH.& Hadley, M. (1990). Malondialdehyde determination as index of lipid peroxidation, *Methods Enzymol* 186: 421-431.

Dwivedi, Vk. , Chandra, KM. , Misra, PC. & Misra, MK. (2005). Effect of vitamin E on platelet enzymatic anti-oxidants in the patients of myocardial infarction, *Indian Journal of Clinical Biochemistry.* 20 (1): 21- 25.

Evangelista, FS., Brum, PC.& Krieger JE. (2003). Duration-controlled swimming exercise training induces cardiac hypertrophy in mice, *Braz J Med Biol Res.*36:1751-1759.

Farshid, AA., Sadeghi-Hashjin, G.& Ferdowsi, HR. (2002). Histopathological studies on the effects of peroxynitrite on the lungs and trachea of rabbits, *Eur Respir J* 20: 1014-1016.

Feki, M., Souissi, M. & Mebazaa, A. (2001). Vitamin E: structure, metabolism, and functions, *Ann Med Interne (Paris).* 152: 384.

Fisher, RA. & Yates, F. (1957). Statistical tables for biological structure and medical research, 5th edition:3.

Freedman, JE. & Keaney, JF. (2001). Vitamin E Inhibition of Platelet Aggregation Is Independent of Antioxidant Activity, *J Nutrition.* 131:374S-377S.

Freedman, JE., Loscalzo, J., Benoit, SE., Valeri, CR., Barnard, MR., and Michelson, AD. (1996). Decreased platelet inhibition by nitric oxide in two brothers with a history of arterial thrombosis, J. Clin. Invest. 97: 979–987.

Gao, WD., Liu, Y.& Marban, E. (1996). Selective effects of oxygen free radicals on excitation-contraction coupling in ventricular muscle. Implications for the mechanism of stunned myocardium, *Circulation* 15;94(10):2597-2604.

Gawaz, M. (2004). Role of platelets in coronary thrombosis and reperfusion of ischemic myocardium, Cardiovascular Research. 61: 498–511.

Ghali, JK. , Liao, Y.& Cooper, RS. (1997). Left Ventricular Hypertrophy in the Elderly, *Am J Geriatr Cardiol.* 6: 38-49.

Gilbert, VA., Zebrowski, EJ. & Chen, AC. (1983).Differential effects of megavitamin E on prostacyclin and thromboxane synthesis in streptozotocin-induced diabetic rats, *Horm Metab Res.* 15: 320.

Gourdin, MG.; Bree, B. & De Kock, M. (2009). The impact of ischaemia-reperfusion on the blood vessel, *Eu J Anaesthesiol.* 26(7):537- 47.

Gurbel, PA. , Serebruany, VL. , Komjathy, S F. , Collins, M E. , Sane, DC. ,Scott , H J., Schlossberg M L. & Herzog WR. (1995). Regional and systemic platelet function is altered by myocardial ischemia-reperfusion, *J Thromb Thrombolysis.* 1: 187-194.

Halestrap, AP., Clarke, SJ.& Javadov, SA. (2004). Mitochondrial permeability transition pore opening during myocardial reperfusion--a target for cardioprotection, *Cardiovasc Res* 61: 372-385.

Hanson, MG., Ozenci, V., Carlsten, MC., Glimelius, BL., Frödin, JE., Masucci, G., Malmberg, KJ.& Kiessling, RV.(2007).A short-term dietary supplementation with high doses of vitamin E increases NK cell cytolytic activity in advanced colorectal cancer patients, *Cancer Immunol Immunother* 56: 973-984.

Hatao, H., Oh-ishi, S., Itoh, M., Leeuwenburgh, C., Ohno, H., Ookawara, T., Kishi, K., Yagyu, H., Nakamura, H.& Matsuoka, T. (2006). Effects of acute exercise on lung antioxidant enzymes in young and old rats, *Mech Ageing Dev.* 127(4):384-390.

Higashi, O. & Kikuchi, Y. (1974). Effects of vitamin E on the aggregation and the lipid peroxidation of platelets exposed to hydrogen peroxide, *Tohoku J Exp Med.* 112: 271.

Hunter EE, editor. (1984) Practical electron microscopy. A beginner's illustrated guide. New York (NY): Praeger Publishers Inc.

Kamat, JP. (2006). Peroxynitrite: a potent oxidizing and nitrating agent, *Indian J Exp Biol.* 44: 436-447.

Karpen, CW., Merola, AJ., Trewyn, RW., Cornwell, DG. & Panganamala, RV. (1981). Modulation of platelet thromboxane A_2 and arterial prostacyclin by dietary vitamin E, *Prostaglandins.* 22: 651.

Kassim, SK.(1997). Determination of Cytosolic Nitrite and Nitrate as Indicators of Nitric Oxide Level in Ovarian Cancer Cells, *CMB.* 4: 1051-1059.

Kim, JS., Jin, Y. &, Lemasters, JJ. (2006). Reactive oxygen species, but not Ca2+ overloading, trigger pH- and mitochondrial permeability transition-dependent death of adult rat myocytes after ischemia-reperfusion, *Am J Physiol Heart Circ Physiol*;290: H2024-H2034.

Kiran, T., Subramanyam, MV. & Asha Devi S. (2004). Swim exercise training and adaptations in the antioxidant defense system of myocardium of old rats: relationship to swim intensity and duration, *Comp Biochem Physiol B Biochem Mol Biol.* 137: 187-196.

Krasavage, WJ. & Terhaar CJ.(1977). d-alpha-Tocopheryl poly(ethylene glycol) 1000 succinate, Acute toxicity, subchronic feeding, reproduction, and teratologic studies in the rat, *J Agric Food Chem* 25: 273-278.

Kwak, HB., Song, W.& Lawler JM. (2006). Exercise training attenuates age-induced elevation in Bax/Bcl-2 ratio, apoptosis, and remodeling in the rat heart, *FASEB J.* 20: 791-793.

Lefer, AM., Campbell, B., Scalia, R. & Lefer, DJ. (1998): Synergism between platelets and neutrophils in provoking cardiac dysfunction after ischemia and reperfusion: role of selectins, *Circulation.* 98: 1322– 8.

Libonati, J., Kendrick, Z.& Houser, R. (2005). Sprint training improves postischemic, left ventricular diastolic performance, *J Appl Physiol.* 99: 2121-2127.

Massberg, S.; Enders, G.; Leiderer, R.; Eisenmenger, S.; Vestweber, D.; Krombach, F. & Messmer, K. (1998). Platelet-Endothelial Cell Interactions During Ischemia/Reperfusion:The Role of P-Selectin, *Blood.* 92:507-515. Matz, RL., de Sotomayor, MA., Schott, C., Stoclet, JC.& Andriantsitohaina, R. (2000). Vascular bed heterogeneity in age-related endothelial dysfunction with respect to NO and eicosanoids, *Br J Pharmacol.* 131: 303-311.

Murohara, T., Ikeda, H., Otsuka, Y., Aoki, M., Haramaki, N., Katoh, A., Takajo ,Y. & Imaizumi, T. (2004). Inhibition of Platelet Adherence to Mononuclear Cells by α-

Tocopherol : Role of P-Selectin, *Circulation*.110:141-148. Murphy, E. & Steenbergen, C. (2008). Mechanisms Underlying Acute Protection From Cardiac Ischemia-Reperfusion Injury, *Physiol Rev* 88 (2): 581-609.

Navarro, A., Gómez, C., Sánchez-Pino, MJ., González, H., Bández, MJ., Boveris, AD.& Boveris, A. (2005).Vitamin E at high doses improves survival, neurological performance, and brain mitochondrial function in aging male mice, *Am J Physiol Regul Integr Comp Physiol* 289: R1392- R1399.

Pignatelli, P., Pulcinelli, FM., Lenti, L., Gazzaniga, PP. & Violi, F. (1999). Vitamin E inhibits collagen-induced platelet activation by plunting hydrogen peroxide, *Arterioscler Thromb Vasc Biol.* 19: 2542.

Pritchard, KA., Karpen, CW., Merola, AJ. & Panganamala, RV. (1982). Influence of dietary vitamin E on platelet thromboxane A_2 and vascular prostacyclin I_2 in rabbit, *Prostaglandins Leukot Med.* 9:373.

Qin, F., Yan, C., Patel, R., Liu, W., Dong, E. (2006).Vitamins C and E attenuate apoptosis, beta-adrenergic receptor desensitization, and sarcoplasmic reticular Ca2+ ATPase downregulation after myocardial infarction, *Free Radic Biol Med* 40: 1827-1842.

Refaat, MRA., El-Nasr, AS., Farrag, HF.& Ayobe, MH. (1989). Plasma libid changes following short term exercise program in rats, *Ain Shams Medical Journal.* 40:515-520.

Ricciarelli, R., Zingg, JM.& Azzi, A. (2002). The 80th anniversary of vitamin E: beyond its antioxidant properties, *Biol Chem* 383: 457-465.

Sheu, SS., Nauduri, D.& Anders, MW. (2006). Targeting antioxidants to mitochondria: a new therapeutic direction, *Biochim Biophys Acta* 1762: 256-265.

Sohal, R J., Arnold, L A.& Sohal, B H. (1990). Age-related changes in antioxidant enzymes and prooxidant generation in tissues of the rat with special reference to parameters in two insect species, *Free Radical Biol Med.* 10:495–500.

Srivastava, KC. (1986). Vitamin E exerts antiaggregatory effects without inhibiting the enzymes of the arachidonic acid cascade in platelets, *Prostaglandins Leukot Med.*21: 177.

Steiner, M. & Anastasi, J. (1976). Vitamin E. An inhibitor of the platelet release reaction, *J Clin Invest.* 57: 732. Tanguy, S., Boucher, F., Besse, S., Ducros, V., Favier, A.& de Leiris, J. (1998).Trace elements and cardioprotection: increasing endogenous glutathione peroxidase activity by oral selenium supplementation in rats limits reperfusion-induced arrhythmias, *J Trace Elem Med Biol.* 12(1):28-38.

Venditti, P., Masullo, P., Di Meo, S.& Agnisola C. (1999). Protection against ischemia-reperfusion induced oxidative stress by vitamin E treatment, *Arch Physiol Biochem.* 107: 27-34.

Wang, G., Liem, DA., Vondriska, TM., Honda, HM., Korge, P., Pantaleon, DM., Qiao, X., Wang, Y., Weiss, JN. &, Ping P. (2005). Nitric oxide donors protect murine myocardium against infarction via modulation of mitochondrial permeability transition, *Am J Physiol Heart Circ Physiol* 288: H1290-H1295.

Xia, Y., Khatchikian, G.& Zweier, J L. (1996). Adenosine Deaminase Inhibition Prevents Free Radical-mediated Injury in the Postischemic Heart, *J Biol Chem.* 271:10096–10102.

Xu, Y. , Huo, Y. ,Toufektsian , MC. , Ramos, SI. , Ma, Y. , Tejani, AD., French, BA. & Yang, Z. (2006). Activated platelets contribute importantly to myocardial reperfusion injury, *Am J Physiol Heart Circ Physiol.* 290: H692- 9.

Yamazaki, K., Miwa, S., Ueda, K., Tanaka, S., Toyokuni, S., Unimonh, O., et al. 2004 Prevention of myocardial reperfusion injury by poly(ADP-ribose) synthetase inhibitor, 3-aminobenzamide, in cardioplegic solution: in vitro study of isolated rat heart model, *Eur J Cardiothorac Surg* 26: 270-275.

Zhou, ZH., Peng, J., Ye, F., Li, NS., Deng, HW.& Li, YJ. (2002). Delayed cardioprotection induced by nitroglycerin is mediated by alphacalcitonin gene-related peptide, *Naunyn Schmiedebergs Arch Pharmacol* 365: 253-259.

Permissions

The contributors of this book come from diverse backgrounds, making this book a truly international effort. This book will bring forth new frontiers with its revolutionizing research information and detailed analysis of the nascent developments around the world.

We would like to thank Umashankar Lakshmanadoss MD, for lending his expertise to make the book truly unique. He has played a crucial role in the development of this book. Without his invaluable contribution this book wouldn't have been possible. He has made vital efforts to compile up to date information on the varied aspects of this subject to make this book a valuable addition to the collection of many professionals and students.

This book was conceptualized with the vision of imparting up-to-date information and advanced data in this field. To ensure the same, a matchless editorial board was set up. Every individual on the board went through rigorous rounds of assessment to prove their worth. After which they invested a large part of their time researching and compiling the most relevant data for our readers. Conferences and sessions were held from time to time between the editorial board and the contributing authors to present the data in the most comprehensible form. The editorial team has worked tirelessly to provide valuable and valid information to help people across the globe.

Every chapter published in this book has been scrutinized by our experts. Their significance has been extensively debated. The topics covered herein carry significant findings which will fuel the growth of the discipline. They may even be implemented as practical applications or may be referred to as a beginning point for another development. Chapters in this book were first published by InTech; hereby published with permission under the Creative Commons Attribution License or equivalent.

The editorial board has been involved in producing this book since its inception. They have spent rigorous hours researching and exploring the diverse topics which have resulted in the successful publishing of this book. They have passed on their knowledge of decades through this book. To expedite this challenging task, the publisher supported the team at every step. A small team of assistant editors was also appointed to further simplify the editing procedure and attain best results for the readers.

Our editorial team has been hand-picked from every corner of the world. Their multi-ethnicity adds dynamic inputs to the discussions which result in innovative outcomes. These outcomes are then further discussed with the researchers and contributors who give their valuable feedback and opinion regarding the same. The feedback is then collaborated with the researches and they are edited in a comprehensive manner to aid the understanding of the subject.

Apart from the editorial board, the designing team has also invested a significant amount of their time in understanding the subject and creating the most relevant covers. They scrutinized every image to scout for the most suitable representation of the subject and create an appropriate cover for the book.

The publishing team has been involved in this book since its early stages. They were actively engaged in every process, be it collecting the data, connecting with the contributors or procuring relevant information. The team has been an ardent support to the editorial, designing and production team. Their endless efforts to recruit the best for this project, has resulted in the accomplishment of this book. They are a veteran in the field of academics and their pool of knowledge is as vast as their experience in printing. Their expertise and guidance has proved useful at every step. Their uncompromising quality standards have made this book an exceptional effort. Their encouragement from time to time has been an inspiration for everyone.

The publisher and the editorial board hope that this book will prove to be a valuable piece of knowledge for researchers, students, practitioners and scholars across the globe.

List of Contributors

Umashankar Lakshmanadoss
Formerly Director, Inpatient Consult Service, Johns Hopkins University School of Medicine, Baltimore, MD Division of Cardiology, Guthrie Clinic, Sayre, PA, USA

Mette Bjerre
The Medical Research Laboratories, Institute of Clinical Medicine, Faculty of Health Sciences, Aarhus University, Denmark

Sadip Pant and Abhishek Deshmukh
University of Arkansas for Medical Sciences, Little Rock, AR, USA

Pritam Neupane
Medical College of Georgia, Augusta, GA, USA

M.P. Kavin Kumar
Department of Internal Medicine, Priya Hospital-Heart and Diabetic Care, Tamil Nadu, India

C.S. Vijayashankar
Apollo Hospitals Greams Road, Chennai, Tamil Nadu, India

Jens Broscheit
Department of Anethesiology, University Clinics of Würzburg, Germany

E.P. Tatarchenko, N.V. Pozdnyakova, O.E. Morozova and E.A. Petrushin
Penza Extension Course Institute for Medical Practitioners, Russia

Ajay Suri, Syed Ahsan and Pascal Meier
The Heart Hospital, University College Hospital, London, UK

Sophia Tincey
North Middlesex Hospital, London, UK

Raveen Naidoo and Nicholas Castle
Durban University of Technology, South Africa

Javier E. Horta and Mahdi Garelnabi
Department of Clinical Laboratory and Nutritional Sciences, University of Massachusetts Lowell, Lowell, MA, USA

Emir Veledar
Emory University School of Medicine Atlanta, GA, USA

Nermine Saleh and Magda Youssef
Faculty of Medicine, Ain Shams University, Physiology Department, Egypt